Maxillofacial Surgery and Craniofacial Deformity - Practices and Updates

Edited by Mazen Ahmad Almasri and Raja Kummoona

Published in London, United Kingdom

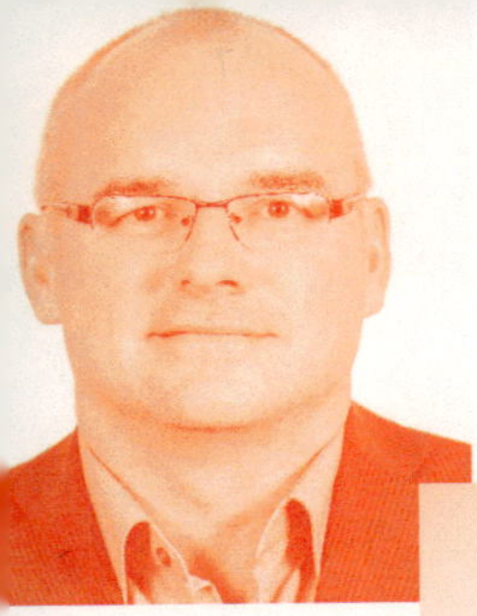
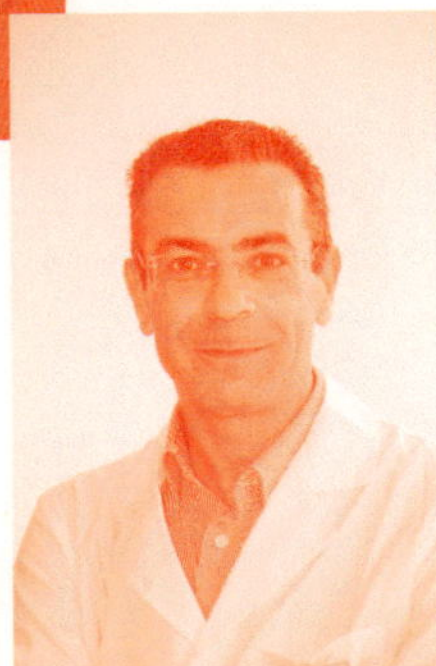
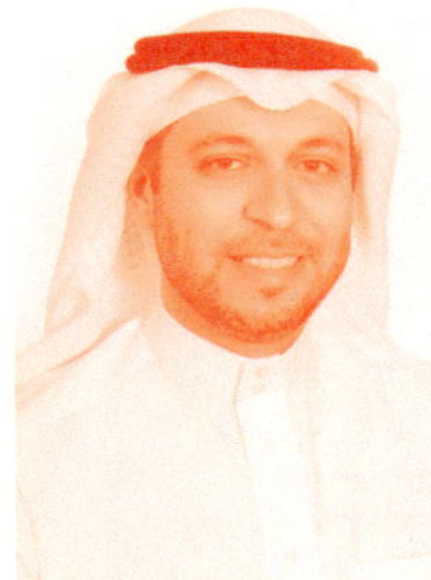
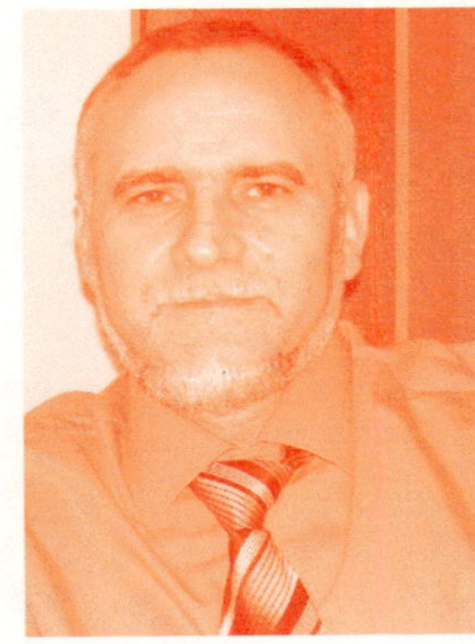
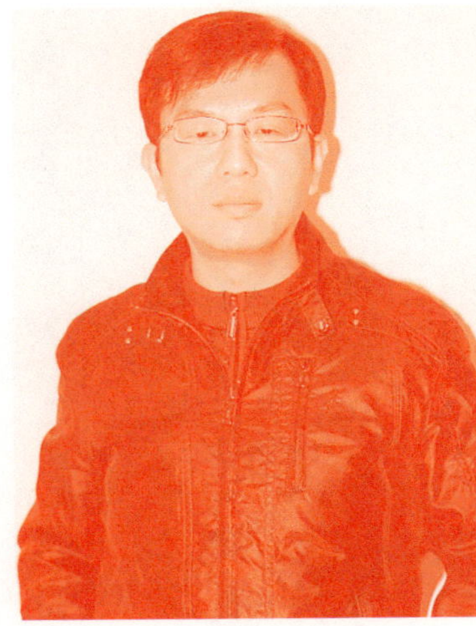
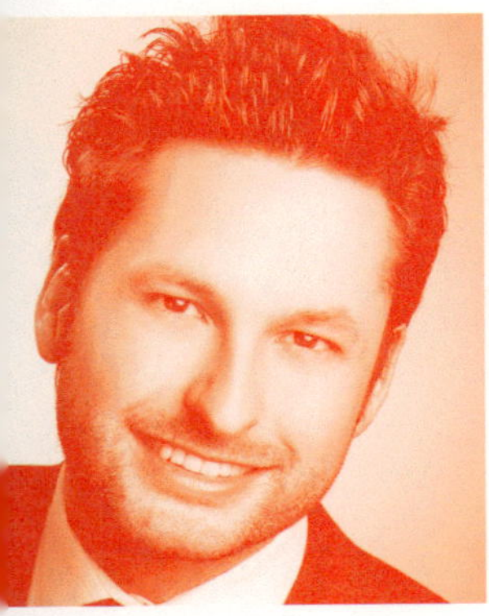
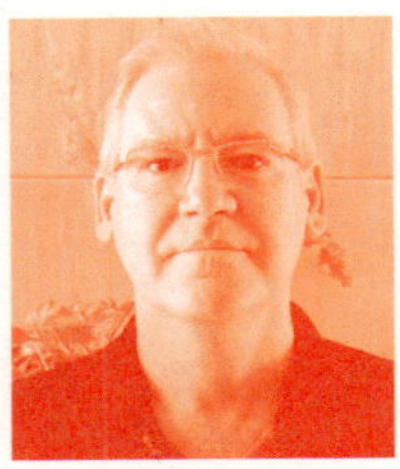

IntechOpen

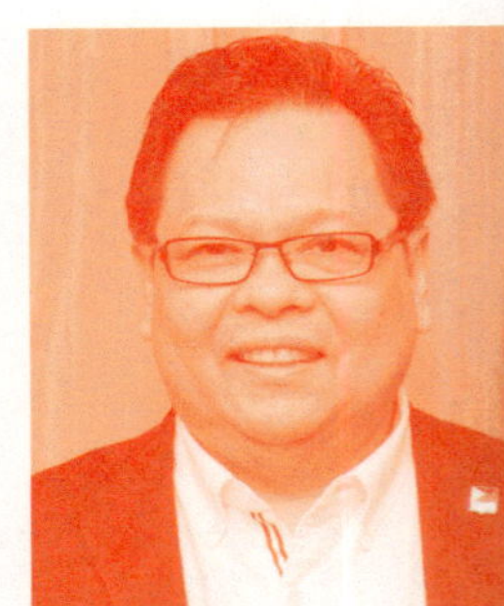
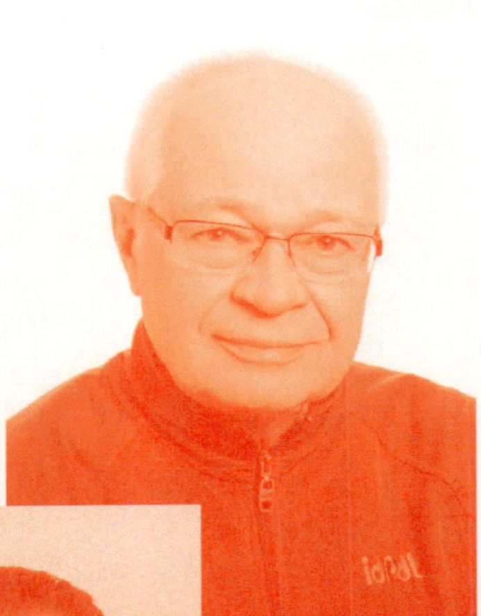
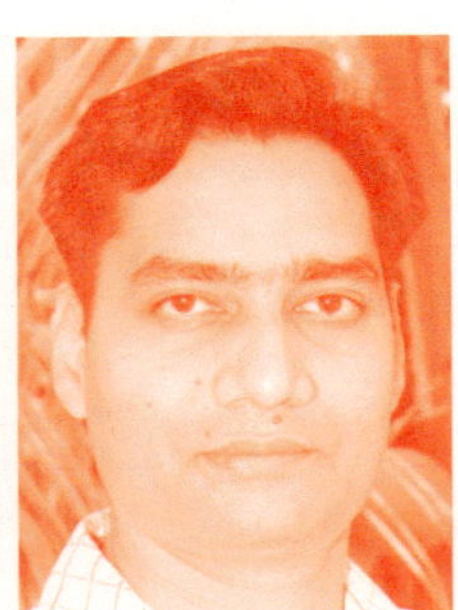
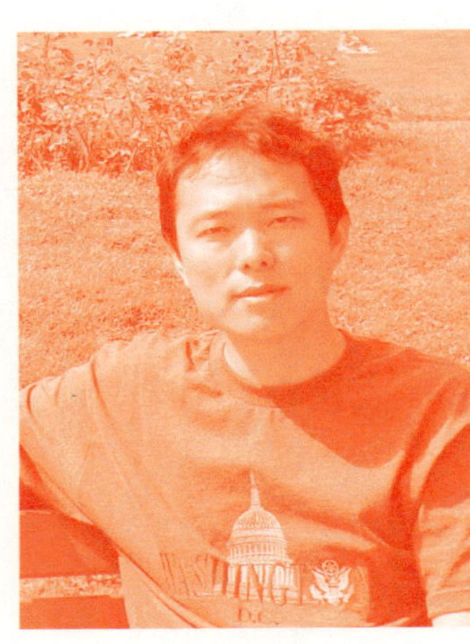
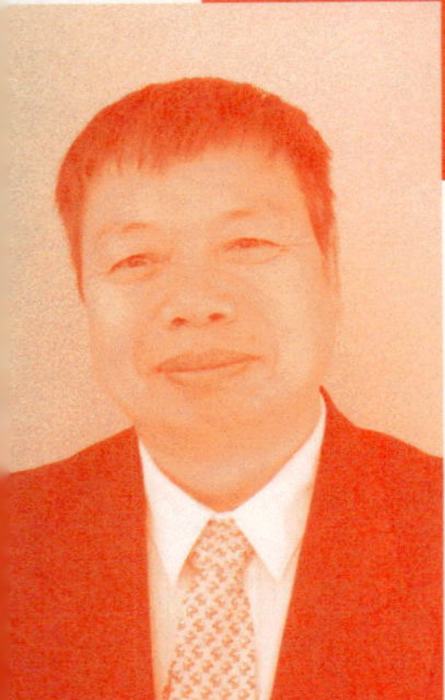
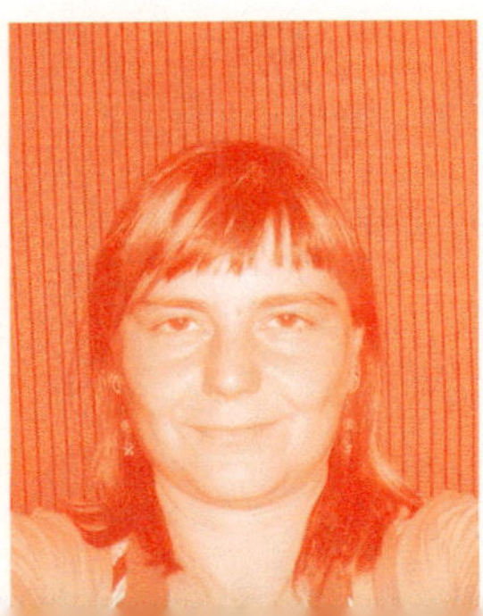

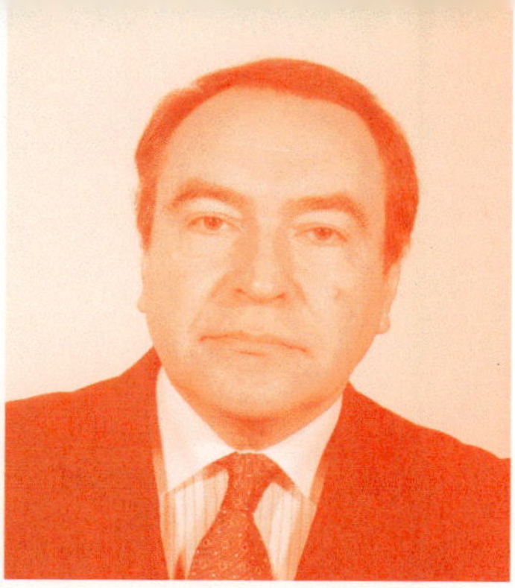
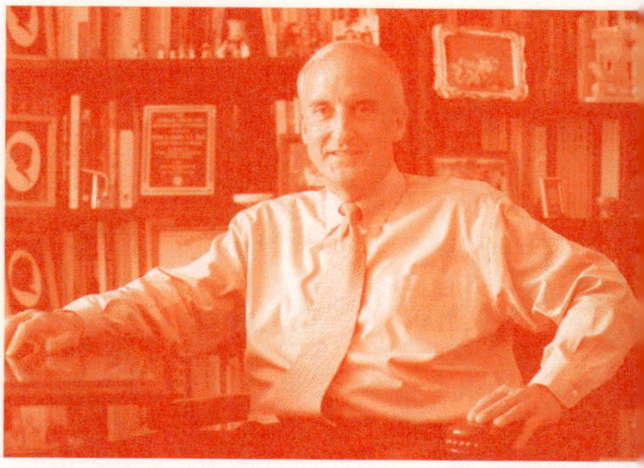
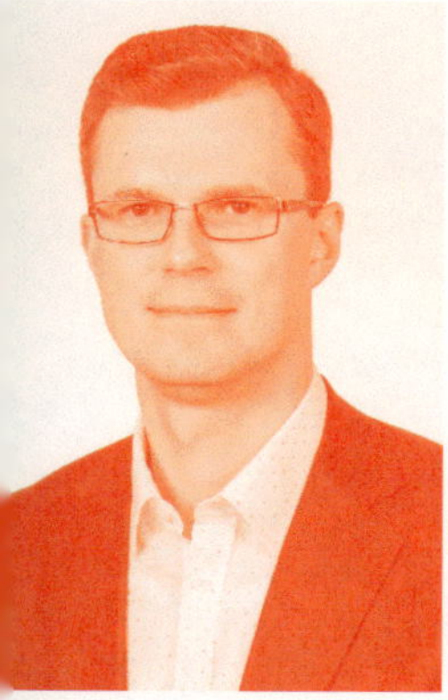
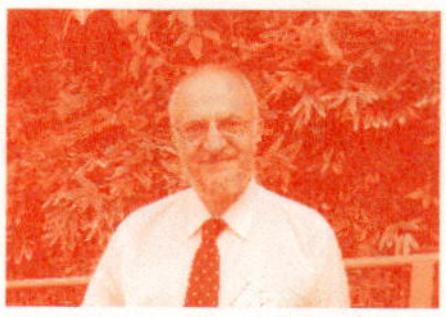
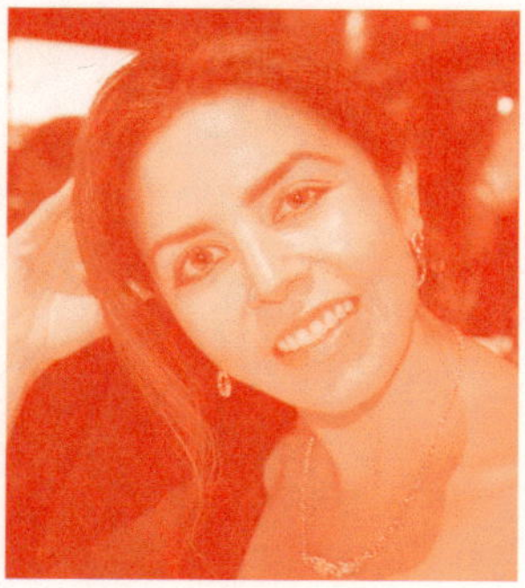

Supporting open minds since 2005

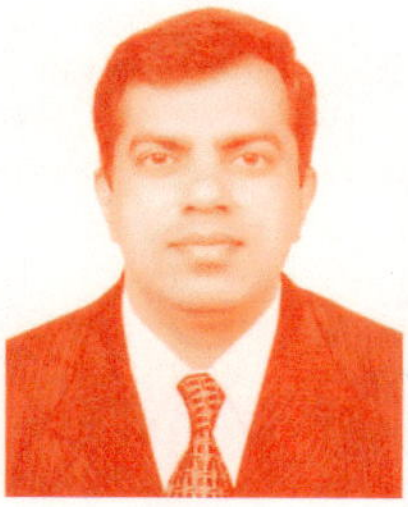
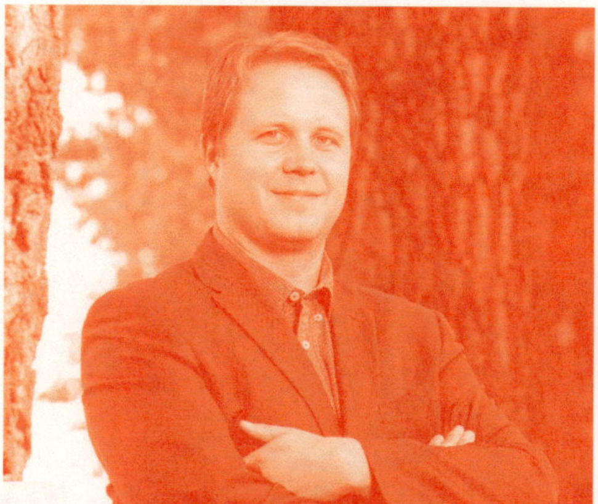
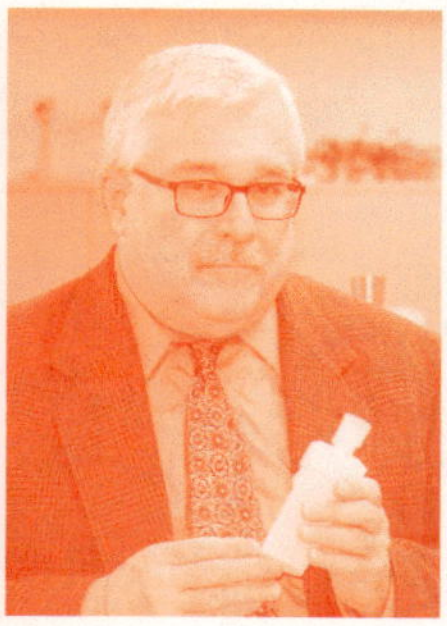
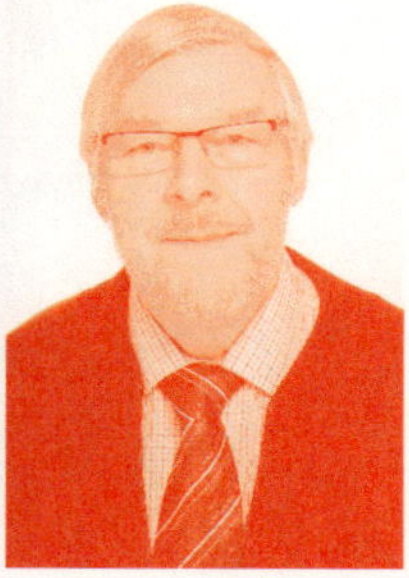
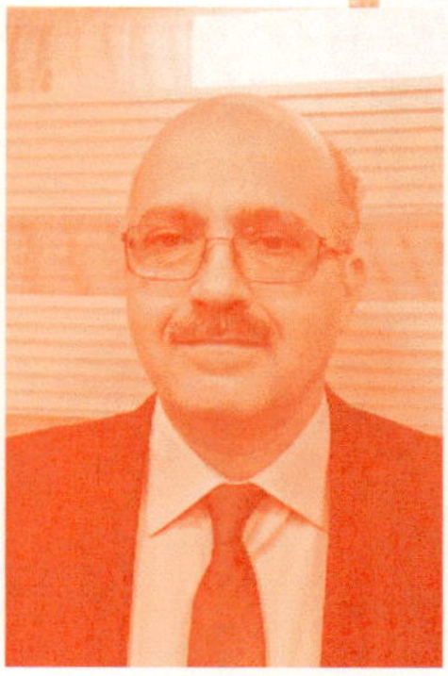
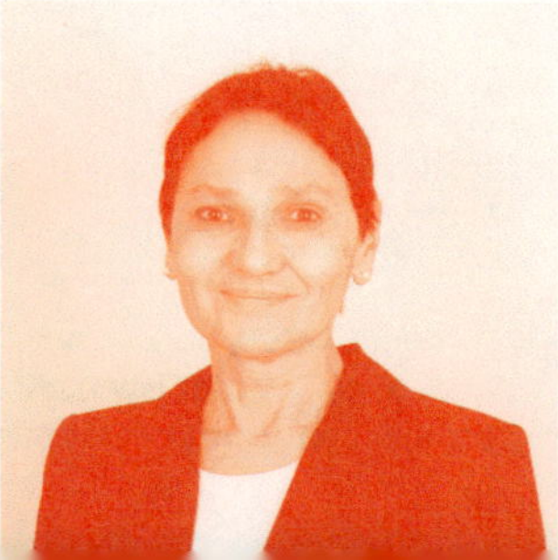
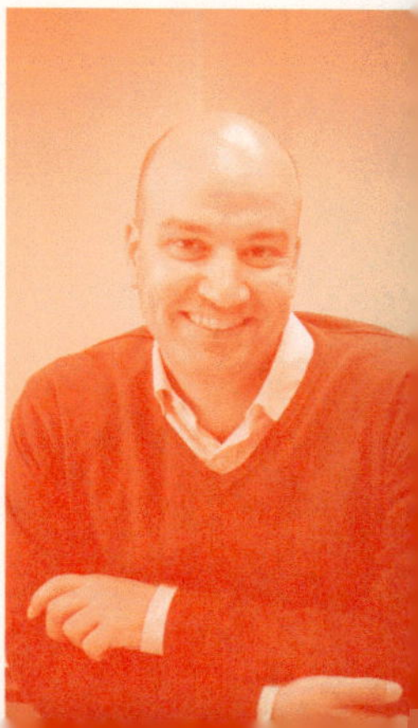

Maxillofacial Surgery and Craniofacial Deformity - Practices and Updates
http://dx.doi.org/10.5772/intechopen.77758
Edited by Mazen Ahmad Almasri and Raja Kummoona

Contributors
Nedeljka Ivkovic, Maja Racic, Marko Blašković, Dorotea Blaskovic, Luiz Avelar, Luciene Menrique Corradi, Naida Hadziabdic, Turker Yucesoy, Ramat Braimah, Dominic Ukpong, Kizito Ndukwe, Takako Sato, Ryota Nakamura, Akio Himejima, Akemi Kusano, Serim Kang, Saori Ohtani, Kentarou Yamada, Junya Aoki, Takeya Yamada, Morio Tonogi, Ahmet Baki, Wilber Edison Bernaola-Paredes, Henrique Cabrini Cabrini Moreira, Raja K Kummoona, Kanako Yamagata, Hiroaki Azaki, Keiichi Yanagawa, Keiji Shinozuka

First published in London, United Kingdom, 2020 by IntechOpen
IntechOpen is the global imprint of INTECHOPEN LIMITED, registered in England and Wales, registration number: 11086078, 7th floor, 10 Lower Thames Street, London, EC3R 6AF, United Kingdom
Printed in Croatia

British Library Cataloguing-in-Publication Data
A catalogue record for this book is available from the British Library

Additional hard and PDF copies can be obtained from orders@intechopen.com

Maxillofacial Surgery and Craniofacial Deformity - Practices and Updates
Edited by Mazen Ahmad Almasri and Raja Kummoona
p. cm.
Print ISBN 978-1-78985-411-4
Online ISBN 978-1-78985-412-1
eBook (PDF) ISBN 978-1-83880-852-5

For EU product safety concerns:
IN TECH d.o.o., Prolaz Marije Krucifikse Kozulić 3, 51000 Rijeka, Croatia, info@intechopen.com or visit our website at intechopen.com.

Meet the editors

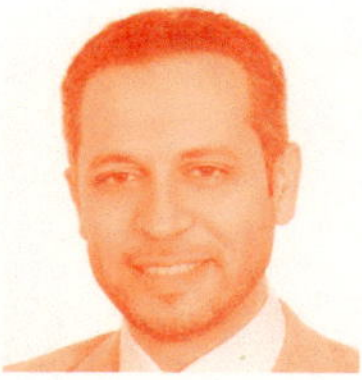

Dr Mazen AJ Almasri is an Associate Professor of Oral Maxillofacial Surgery at the King Abdulaiz University, Faculty of Dentistry, Saudi Arabia. He graduated from KAU in 2002 with an honors degree, then pursued his clinical training of OMFS at McGill University, (Montreal, Quebec, Canada) where he became an active fellow of the Royal College of Canada in 2009, achieved his Masters degree (2010), the Implantology and Reconstruction Fellowship (2010), and was an active diplomate of the American Board of OMFS (2011). Dr Almasri's passion toward advancing the health care and medical education continued through teaching undergraduate and postgraduate trainees, and pursuing publication of papers and text books.

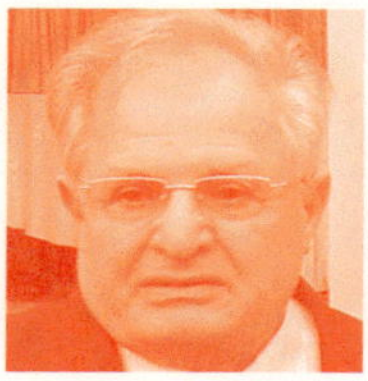

Professor Raja Kummoona is a Fellow of the Royal College of Surgeons of England (FDSRCS), Emeritus professor of Maxillofacial Surgery of Iraqi Board for Medical Specializations, Fellow Royal Society of Medicine, Research Fellow Royal College of Surgeons of England from 1975 to 1977, President of Iraqi Dental Society (1977-1985), Registrar of Primary FDSRCS in Iraq (1985-1990), the most distinguished professor of the University of Baghdad (1991-1992), one of 40 top scientist in Iraq awarded a gold medal for 3 years (2000-2002) by presidential celebration. He has had many publications and contribution to science by advocating many surgical procedures and research in cancer surgery and flap reconstruction, TMJ surgery and maxillofacial injuries, orbit tumors and injuries, missile war injuries of the face with advancing surgery of war injuries of the face worldwide. He has contributed to research in cancer and has developed post graduate studies in maxillofacial surgery in Iraq. He is the Editor of *Neck Dissection, Clinical Application and Recent Advances* (February, 2012, IntechOpen), *Surgical Reconstruction of the Temporomandibular Joint* (2013), Germany, *Disease of the TMJ, Surgical reconstruction, clinical & experimental studies* (April, 2014, Science PG), *Missile war injuries of the face, maxillofacial injuries in road traffic* (book published by Science PG, 2014), and *Jaw lymphoma and orofacial tumors* (2015, published by Science PG), *Bone grafting, recent advances with special reference to craniomaxillofacial surgery* (December, 2018, IntechOpen), *Craniofacial deformity and normal variations of jaws relationship* (OMICS International). He is a member of the editorial board of 15 international distinguished journals, President of Society of Iraqi Maxillofacial Surgery, a Founder member of the International Society of Head Neck Trauma, 2015, London, and Chairman of the Department of Maxillofacial Surgery, College of Dentistry, University of Baghdad 1982-2000. He is a member of the Council of College of Dentistry (1975-2000), Founder and Chairman council of Maxillofacial Surgery, Iraqi Board for Medical Specializations (1993-2010). He has about 129 papers published and is an eminent figure in craniofacial surgery in the Middle East.

Contents

Preface

Mazen Ahmad Almasri

Oral and maxillofacial surgery is a dynamic specialty that is evolving and progressively advancing to manage deformities of the face, cranium, oral cavity, jaws, and neck.

It is well known that diagnosis and plan management are modifiable based on the patient status, diagnostic tools, available resources, and man power.

This is clearer when considering the current status of COVID-19, which has introduced a totally new approach for all patients.

This book covers topics including wisdom teeth, impacted teeth, orthognathic malalignment, facial deformities, TMJ diseases, and the social and psychological considerations.

The current health situation has made the preparation and finalization of this textbook even more complicated that it already was. It wouldn't have been possible without a collaborative effort. During the last year, a lot of medical events took place, and passing through the quarantine of COVID-19, the spirit was not taken away from finalizing this book project. I hope that this book will benefit the readers in the field of OMFS and craniofacial deformity and provide another view and insight of OMF deformities, diagnosis, and management.

Mazen Ahmad Almasri
King Abdulaziz University,
Saudi Arabia

Raja Kummoona

The topic of craniofacial deformity is very interesting and difficult topic covering malformation and deformity of the cranium and facial skeleton.

In this book we describe the foundation, establishment, progress, and advances of craniofacial surgery. In the past centuries, Hippocrate, Sushurta, and the advocation of Le Fort III osteotomy for reconstruction of Curzon disease by Sir Harold Gillies and followed by Paul Tessier established the first time his technique for correction of craniofacial malformation and deformity in the 1960s.

One of the great advances in craniofacial surgery include the advocation of penicillin by Sir Alexander Fleming at St Marys Hospital, London during the Second World War.

The most exciting progress and advancement in craniofacial surgery was the application of bone graft and distraction osteogenesis and refinement of instrumentation to facilitate the surgical procedures.

The advancement extended to radiological tools including plain X-ray, CT Scan with 3 dimensions, MRI, ultrasound, and endoscopy. The ultrasound was used to detect the uterus during pregnancy and carried into the uterus for uterine surgery by endoscopy for correction of cleft lip and palate, facial clefts and Pierre Robin syndrome.

Further advancement includes work by Kenneth E Sayler in the 1970s by his operation by advancement of frontal-orbital block in children to let the brain and skull to grow without effect of cranial sutures.

The section on craniofacial deformity surgeries also contains an important chapter dealing with deformity of the craniofacial skeleton by traumatic injuries. This chapter is very interesting because it deals with the deformity of the facial skeleton and its management.

Two further interesting chapters of this book deal with cleft lip and palate, and haemangioma of the nasal septum.

I would like to extend my thanks to Andrea Koric, commissioning editor of IntechOpen, without her kind effort we could not have produced this valuable book and special thanks and gratitude to Sara Debeuc, author service manager, for her outstanding effort in preparation of this valuable book.

Raja Kummoona
Council of Maxillofacial Surgery,
Iraqi Board for Medical Specialization,
Baghdad, Iraq

Section 1

Craniofacial Deformity Surgeries

Chapter 1

Prologue: Foundation and Progress of Craniofacial Surgery of Deformity and Malformation

Raja Kummoona

1. Introduction

Surgery of craniofacial malformation and deformity is a surgical subspecialty that deals with acquired and congenital deformity of the skull and facial skeleton, including the orbits, midface, and jaws.

The history of craniofacial surgery is not new but began with ancient humans drilling holes in the cranial vault (trephination).

In Europe, and especially in France, 40 out of 120 prehistoric skulls were found with drill holes in the skulls. This technique is currently practiced to reduce intracranial pressure and the evacuation of supradural hematoma from the middle meningeal arteries [1, 2].

Craniofacial anomalies have been known throughout history and both Hippocrates and Homer have touched upon the subject. Surgery was possible with the invention of general anesthesia in the mid-nineteenth century and was helped later with the discovery of penicillin by Sir Alexander Fleming of St. Mary's Hospital, Paddington, London, during the Second World War.

Surgeons like Sir Harold Gillies (UK), Hippolyte Morestin (France), and Jan F. Esser (Netherland) were pioneering the specialties of plastic surgery while dealing with war-injured soldiers [3].

In ancient times, reconstructive craniofacial procedures of the soft tissue were performed to reconstruct the nose or ears. Sushruta and other Indian doctors were practicing reconstruction of noses and ear lobes in 600 BC [2].

In India during Sushruta's time, it was common practice for criminals to have their noses amputated because the procedure was considered to be a symbol of reputation and respect. Groups of potters known as Koomas developed a technique of nasal reconstruction to help people with these problems [4].

In Iraq during the Iraqi/Iranian War (1980–1988), young soldiers who avoided front line duty were punished by the Saddam regime by cutting part of their ears or making a symbol on their forehead. This prevented doctors from repairing the created defect and deformity; it was a very depressing procedure for young people and many of them attempted suicide.

Gaspare Tagliacozzi of Bologna was a genius surgeon, and in 1597 was chosen to reconstruct a deformed nose. He did reconstruction of the nose by elevating the pedicle bicipital arm flap as tube pedicle and mobilizing the flap for reconstruction of the nose deformity. This technique required 14 days of immobilization of the arm to attach the face, followed by division and inset of the flap from the arm [5].

The author believes that this technique was the first to use the tube pedicle flap in reconstructive surgery.

Advancements in craniofacial and maxillofacial surgery have been more recently carried out by great surgeons like Paul Tessier, Hugo Obwegeser, Norman Rowe, and Joseph Converse.

Craniofacial surgery formally developed in 1967 after a meeting of well-known international surgeons with Paul Tessier because of pressure on him from French plastic surgeons. Tessier requested them to observe and follow up his cases and to recognize his work on craniofacial deformities at Foch hospital in Paris, where the meeting took place.

Norman Rowe and J.C. Mustardé from Britain, Joseph Converse from the United States, Hugo Obwegeser from Switzerland, and Zur Hausen from Germany were members of the group who spent 2 weeks in Foch hospital examining, observing and following up on 50 of Tessier's cases. Most cases were comprised of poor people from Italy. After 2 weeks Paul Tessier ask the invited committee am I entitled to practice this kind of subspecialties, all of them recognized him pioneered by a man who was recognized as the master of craniofacial surgery. This story was related to the author by Professor Hugo Obwegeser in 1981 during his first visit to Baghdad as my guest.

Paul Tessier made a revolutionary approach to the surgery of deformed skulls and orbital skeletons and was considered to be an expert in this field.

The outstanding pioneering work of Paul Tessier emerged as new specialties of craniofacial surgery. Hugo Obwegeser performed his first Le Fort I osteotomy of the maxilla and sagittal split osteotomy of the ascending ramus of the mandible for correction of the malformation of jaw relationship in 1960. He did this by advancing, pushing back, or rotating the lower jaw for correction of Class III and II skeletal jaw deformities and open bite. The lower jaw was mobilized by pushing backward and forward or rotating the lower jaw to correct the open bite, and a downward movement of the maxilla and application of bone graft in the gap were created by this procedure.

Paul Tessier spent a year training in Rocks down house in Britain with the great British surgeon Sir Harold Gillies. Sir Harold's nurse asked Sir Harold to correct her face, which was deformed because of Crouzon disease. He performed the first Le Fort III operation by advancing the face forward; however, 2 weeks later she relapsed and Sir Harold said he would never repeat the procedure.

Tessier was watching the operation; he learned the technique and studied the failure points of Sir Harold Gillies' procedure. Tessier discovered that by using a bone graft inserted in the gaps created by Gillies' osteotomy through Le Fort III operation it would make the skeleton more stable and free from relapse; these observations contributed to the success of Tessier's technique.

After the Second World War, Sir Harold Gillies expanded the field of congenital malformation. In 1949 he performed the first Le Fort III osteotomy based on facial injuries, which was discovered by French surgeon René Le Fort in 1901.

In the past there was a great deal of controversy regarding the complicated surgery of craniofacial deformities as advocated by Tessier; an operation time of up to 16–18 h and blindness were reported. Kenneth E. Salyer in the mid-1970s advocated less complicated surgery by advancing a frontal-orbital block in children and letting the brain and skull grow and operate without the pressure of cranial sutures [6].

One advantage of craniofacial surgery is the prenatal diagnosis of pre-pediatrics malformation by ultrasound, such as a cleft palate, Pierre Robin syndrome, and facial cleft and the possibilities of using intrauterine microsurgery [1].

The exciting progress in craniofacial surgery by using the bone grafting and distraction technique and advancement of radiological diagnostic tools such as ultrasound and three-dimensional CT scanning and MRI have advanced the design of instrumentation for this type of surgery.

Paul Tessier in 1976 classified facial clefts as neither based on theory nor on embryological definition but on an observation made during clinical examination and operative dissection. These clefts were distributed both around the orbit and eyelids and around the lips and maxilla, and certain clefts are common to these two regions; the cleft of soft tissue and bony clefts do not always exactly coincide [6].

Cooperation is required between the orthodontist and the craniomaxillofacial surgeon during different phases of treatment. The treatment plan starts with the orthodontist who aligns the teeth followed by surgical correction after proper planning, which may be followed by orthodontic treatment for final alignment of the teeth and occlusion.

The distraction technique was advocated by a genius Russian orthopedic surgeon Ilizarof [7] for the elongation of short limbs in children and this technique was later applied to the lower jaw with first arch deformity by McCarthy et al. [8].

Distraction is defined as the process of generating new bone by stretching distraction osteogenesis, traction on living stimulate, and maintaining regeneration and growth by inducing a proliferation of precursor cells. This is defined as neoformed bone and adjacent soft tissue after gradual and controlled displacement of fragment bone and adjacent tissue after gradual and controlled displacement of bone fragment obtained by surgical osteotomy [9].

The distraction technique passes through three phases: the surgical phase, the latent period phase, and the consolidation phase. The most critical phase is the latent period phase. An experimental study was conducted on rabbits to understand the cellular changes associated with the distraction technique. This was achieved by using a bilateral distractor. The hand bone lengthening apparatus was adjusted with 1.5-mm Kirschner wire and was passed through both mandibular bodies. Rhythmic distraction of both corpectomies of the bone using an osteotome was carried out at a rate of 1 mm/day at a rhythm of 0.5 mm twice daily, preceded by a latent period of 7 days. The period for distraction lasted 10 days and an immediate postoperative antibiotic of 1 mL/10-kg IM penicillin streptomycin was prescribed once daily. The segments were held by an external fixator for 6 weeks until consolidation was completed. Bone regeneration was evaluated radiologically for periods of 2 weeks, 4 weeks, and 6 weeks. At the end of the experiment a length of 10 mm was achieved.

Histological examination of the distracted jaw showed mature bone trabeculae in the fibrovascular zone and mesenchymal stem cells with heavy fibroblasts oriented with distraction tension, with blood vessels oriented in the same direction. These changes occurred due to the effect of platelet growth factor (PGF), which was released from platelets from bone marrow of osteotomized bone. Newly formed trabeculae lined by a chain of osteoblasts was also noticed.

Bone regeneration by distraction osteogenesis is a highly complicated and organized process. In the above experiment bone regeneration was observed during distraction based on the pattern of a membranous type of bone proceeded by formation of granulation tissue and release of PGF and mesenchymal stem cells from the bone marrow of osteotomized bone segments and from the overlying periosteum [9].

Bone grafting plays another important role in the successful technique of craniofacial surgery and is considered an important factor in advanced craniofacial surgery by inserting a bone graft in the site of osteotomy to prevent relapse. This might be used in orbital reconstruction and skull defects.

Bone grafting is an interesting topic practiced by craniomaxillofacial surgeons. It is a surgical technique used to fix a problem by using transplanted bone to repair and build or replace missing bone, for example lost pieces of bone caused by a road traffic accident or in post-traumatic missile war injuries or after tumor surgery, by filling the gap of osteotomized bone in craniomaxillofacial surgery and orthopedic surgery. The most common type of bone graft practiced by the author is an autogenous cortico-cancellous type or a cancellous type of bone, with the donor area being the iliac crest [10].

Bone grafting is possible because bone tissue can regenerate completely once the space is provided for it to grow as natural bone.

Bone grafting is a complicated technique requiring highly experienced surgeons with high skill and knowledge of the pathology of bone grafting. The greatest advances in bone grafting occurred during the last four or five decades.

The mechanism of bone grafting was not fully understood by most surgeons and cases of failed procedures were reported. Recently experimental studies on rabbits were conducted by reconstructing the mandible by bone graft from the iliac crest of rabbit after excision of a piece of bone from the mandible. The aim was to study and understand the cellular changes that occur between the free bone graft and the recipient stump of bone of the mandible. Cellular changes were tested in three stages of bone formation after 2 weeks, 4 weeks, and 8 weeks.

It was observed that the cytological changes of bone grafting showed the formation of granulation tissue with mesenchymal stem cells derived from bone marrow of boney segments of the mandible and from the periosteum and covering muscle with release of PGF with large numbers of fibroblasts and tiny small blood vessels. Osteoblast was noticed with chondrocyte and osteoid tissue [11, 12].

It was concluded from experimental studies and research on distraction and bone grafting that cellular changes that occur in bone grafting and distraction with these different surgical techniques are the same, with the presence and release of PGF and mesenchymal stem cells. The only differences are the distraction caused by expansion stress of the periosteum and muscles and the bone graft by rigid fixation, and decortication of both graft and stump of the bones [12].

Another revolutionary work was carried out by David Poswillo in 1974, [13]. He presented his experimental studies on *Macaca irus* monkeys by reconstructing the temporomandibular joint (TMJ) by costal-chondral graft to the damaged TMJ to restore growth of the destroyed condyle. In 1986, Raja Kummoona [14] performed his technique for the reconstruction of the TMJ by using his chondral-osseous graft instead of the costal-osseous graft and supported his work by experimental studies on rabbits. He concluded that graft can grow, repair, and remodel the TMJ due to the presence of mesenchymal stem cells in the graft. This technique has an endogenous mechanism for growth. Kummoona's technique was designed for the reconstruction of first arch syndrome and damaged condyle in ankylosis and hypoplastic condyle for restoring midface growth and length.

It is hoped that this introduction presents the author's views on the history and advancements made in craniofacial surgery during the last five decades.

Author details

Raja Kummoona
Council of Maxillofacial Surgery, Iraqi Board for Medical Specialization, Baghdad, Iraq

*Address all correspondence to: raja_kummoona@hotmail.com

References

[1] Barr JS, Hazem A. The history of craniofacial plastic surgery and modern day pediatric craniofacial reconstruction. Academic Journal of Pediatrics & Neonatology. 2016;**1**(3):AJPN.MS.ID555563

[2] Restok R. Fixing the Brain Mysteries of the Mind. Washington DC, USA: National Geographic Society; 2000

[3] European Society of Craniofacial Surgery. History of Craniofacial Surgery. 2019. Available from: http://www.escfs.org/index.php?=history-cfs

[4] Dwivedi G, Dwivedi S. History of Medicine: Sushruta, the Clinician Teacher Par Excellence. National Informatics Center; 2007

[5] Gnudi MT, Webster JP. The Life and Time of Gaspare Tagliacozzi. New York: Herbert Reichner; 1950

[6] Tessier CA, Mustarde JC, Sayler KE. Symposium on Plastic Surgery in the Orbital Region. St. Louis: CV Mosby; 1976

[7] Ilizarov GA. The principles of the ilizarov method. Bulletin of the Hospital for Joint Diseases Orthopaedic Institute. 1988;**48**(1):1-11

[8] McCarthy JG, Staffenberg DA, Wood RJ, Cutting CB, Grayson BH, Thorne CH. Introduction of an intraoral bone lengthening device. Plastic and Reconstructive Surgery. 1955;**96**(4):978-981

[9] Kummoona R, Jassim AM. Distraction technique of lower jaw on rabbit, experiment studies research. Journal of Stem Cell and Regenerative Biology. 2017;**3**(2):158-162

[10] Kummoona R. Reconstruction of the mandible by bone graft and metal prosthesis. Journal of Craniofacial Surgery. 2009;**20**(4):1100-1107

[11] Kummoona R et al. Reconstruction of lower jaw by iliac bone graft, experimental studies on rabbit and the role of mesenchymal stem cells. Journal of Stem Cell and Regenerative Biology. 2018;**4**(1):20-24

[12] Kummoona R. Distraction osteogenesis and bone grafting in orthopedic and maxillofacial surgery, role of mesenchymal stem cells. EC Orthopaedics. 2019;**10**:2

[13] Poswillo DE. Biological reconstruction of mandibular joint. British Journal of Oral Surgery. 1987;**25**:100-104

[14] Kummoona R. Kummoona chondro-osseous graft, good substitute to condylar growth center and for correction of facial deformity in children. Archives of Otolaryngology and Rhinology. 2017;**3**(3):098-102

Chapter 2

Surgical Approach of Cleft Lip/Palate Patients: The Brazilian Experience

Henrique Cabrini Moreira and Wilber Bernaola-Paredes

Abstract

Cleft lip/palate (CL/P) are among the most common birth defects around the world with a prevalence of 1.43:1000 live births. Other studies have shown that the frequency is approximately 1 in 600/700 live births and correction involves prolonged treatment over many years. A variety of surgical techniques and modifications have been described regarding cleft lip and palate (CLP) treatment 2. However, patients still seem to have concerns about their facial appearance, especially related to the cleft deformity. The self-perceived improvement in facial appearance following treatment had a strong positive influence on quality of life and patient satisfaction compared to other functional or treatment-related factors. Depending on the cleft type and severity, as well as treatment outcome, important functions like eating, speech, appearance, and maxillary growth may be impaired. This can affect patients social-emotional functioning and self-esteem resulting in a lower health-related quality of life.

Keywords: cleft lip, cleft palate, spina, surgical approach, palatoplasty, cheiloplasty, seasonal factor, Brazilian experience

1. Cleft lip/palate: general considerations

Cleft lip/palate (CL/P) are among the most common birth defects around the world with a prevalence of 1.43:1000 live births. Other studies have shown that the frequency is approximately 1 in 600/700 live births and correction involves prolonged treatment over many years [1, 2].

A variety of surgical techniques and modifications have been described regarding cleft lip and palate (CLP) treatment [2]. However, patients still seem to have concerns about their facial appearance, especially related to the cleft deformity. The self-perceived improvement in facial appearance following treatment had a strong positive influence on quality of life and patient satisfaction compared to other functional or treatment-related factors [1–3].

The multifactorial threshold model is one of the well-established models for describing the etiology of CL/P, in which statements, the malformations result from factors such as genetic predisposition and exogenous factors like maternal malnutrition, low intake of folic acid, teratogens including drugs and alcohol, viruses, and maternal age [1].

Other studies considerated seasonal influence [1] and they considered that it was reasonable to expect the orofacial clefts may show seasonal variations due to indirect factors such as: maternal malnutrition and low intake of folic acid, and other direct factors such as temperature, intensity of ultraviolet light exposure, use of fertilizers and pesticides in agriculture, and infectious disease cycles.

Depending on the cleft type and severity, as well as treatment outcome, important functions like eating, speech, appearance, and maxillary growth may be impaired. This can affect patients social-emotional functioning and self-esteem resulting in a lower health-related quality of life [3].

The professional's opinion is influenced by training and experience and they may influence patients and parents' perception of the need for treatment. Professionals could also be considered as part of the community with distinct characteristics deriving from their medical background [3–7].

2. Epidemiological profile in Brazilian and Latin-American community in cleft/lip palate

In Brazil [1] and part of Latin-American community, epidemiological studies demonstrated that incidence of CL/P episodes varies from 0.19 to 1.4/1000 births. Approximately 65–70% of cleft lip with or without cleft palate (CLP) and 40–70% of cleft palate only (CP) were isolated defects and the remaining related to syndromic clefts.

A systematic review discussing the issue have also demonstrated that its incidence varies according to gender, 2:1 being the ratio of males to females for cleft lip and palate and 1:2 the approximate ratio of male to female for isolated CP, as well as unilateral clefts are more common than bilateral clefts, and of the unilateral cases of non-syndromic clef lip and palate, left-sided cleft lips occur more frequently than right-sided cleft lips [8].

3. Cleft lip/palate classification

The anatomical, physiological, and pathological understanding of cleft lip/palate is basis for team surgery such as oral and maxillofacial surgeon, plastic surgeon, dentists, and clinicians for enhancing a better clinical approach. Accurate and correct diagnosis is translated through these fundamentals. Thus, patients with cleft lip-palate require a thorough knowledge of all the complexity that affects them.

Whether from the classification system based on anatomical-clinical or embryological issues to the therapeutic models.

Therefore, in this part of the chapter we will discuss the most commonly used classifications in these patients.

3.1 Clefts lip/palate

Regarding treatment of patients with cleft lip/palate (CL/P), Spina [9] modified one of the worldwide used classification in 1973 in order to make a classification easier to understand, simpler to teach, more manageable to memorize, and more applicable to interdisciplinary and international communication.

He had modified previous classification, referred to an anatomical structure placed in the hard palate, the incisive foramen. Accordingly, Spina renamed group 1 as pre-foraminal clefts, group 2 as trans-foraminal, and group 3 as post-foraminal clefts.

These units are further subdivided into unilateral, bilateral, complete, and incomplete, as visualized in **Table 1**.

Silva-Filho [11] adding a sub-classification in the clefts trans-foraminal, named as median type, which is not present in the Spina classification, describes another classification.

Group I	Pre-foraminal	Unilateral Bilateral	Total Partial
Group II	Trans-foraminal	Unilateral Bilateral	
Group III	Post-foraminal	Total Partial	
Group IV	Facial clefts		

Adapted from: Ref. [10].

Table 1.
Cleft and lip/palate classification by Spina [10].

4. Cheiloplasty or plastic lip surgery

The basic statement of lip cleft correction surgery is to approach the edges of the non-tensioned wound. To achieve this result, different techniques are then used from local flaps for the closure of the labial cleft.

The cheiloplasty is ideally recommended to be performed at 3 months of age. There is no need to perform interventions prior to this age, because it has already proven in the literature that will not bring superior esthetic gains and; therefore, due to cicatricial fibrosis, in future in other secondary surgeries, the tissue will be a more difficult for manipulation with less tissue remaining for posterior any necessary esthetic procedure.

Thus, primary cheiloplasty is restricted to only one definitive procedure at 3 months of age, without any previous intervention to "facilitate" the closure of the fissure, shown in **Figure 1**.

4.1 Unilateral cheiloplasty

The clefts can be presented in different ways. For this reason, the surgical planning must be individualized for each patient. As above described, surgery for the lip cleft, whether unilateral or bilateral, should be performed as of the 10th week of life and referred to rule of 10 (hemoglobin 10 mg/dl, 10 weeks of life, and 10 pounds—corresponds to around 4.5–5 kg) [12–14].

The purpose of this surgery is to relocate the surrounded labial tissues: skin, orbicularis muscle of the lip and mucosa. Indeed, for removing the hypoplastic tissue from the margin of the cleft (specifically, could be or not performed, and it will

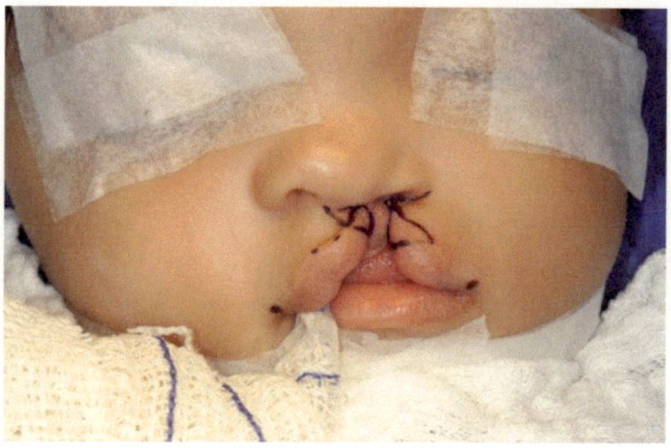

Figure 1.
Patient with unilateral left lip cleft who will submitted to Millard technique. Author: Case report from Oral and Maxillofacial Department of "Defeitos da Face" Medical Center, Sao Paulo, Brazil.

depend how huge the cleft is shown and the addressed tissue will be found). Several techniques are described in the literature for the closure of unilateral lip cleft.

One of the most common used techniques currently is Millard's (seen in **Figure 1**). This technique has the great advantage of allowing that when the tissue advances are performed, they are positioned in the natural contours of the lip and nose (**Figures 1–3**).

4.2 Palatoplasty of plastic palate surgery

The primary surgical correction of the hard and/or soft palate cleft known, as palatoplasty is the surgical procedure for the anatomical, functional and esthetic reconstruction of this structure. Usually, the cleft palate is submitted to surgical treatment between 9 and 12 months of born. Nowadays, the main challenge is to achieve an intervention that minimizes speech changes, without compromising maxillofacial growth [15, 16].

In the current literature, there is still no consensus as which would be the best and accurate technique for correction of the cleft palate. There are a number of techniques of palatoplasty, in which surgeons choose their approach according to their established precepts and experiences.

The choice of the most appropriate technique is an important factor for the clinical success in order to correct this born malformation. Therefore, the surgeon should know which one presents more benefits with lower complications as much as possible [17].

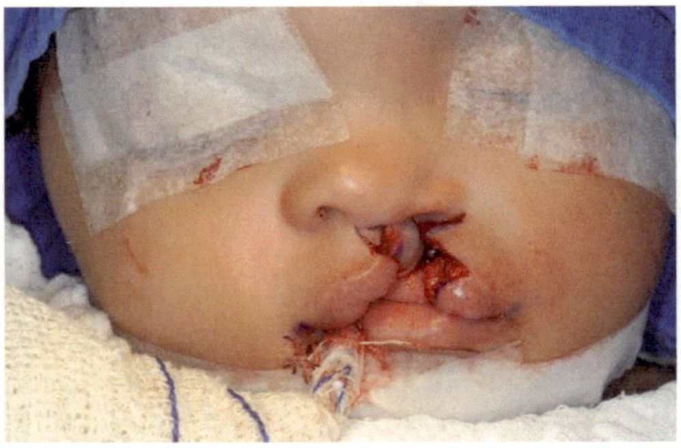

Figure 2.
Free-tension flaps for lip cleft correction. Author: Case report from Oral and Maxillofacial Department of "Defeitos da Face" Medical Center, Sao Paulo, Brazil.

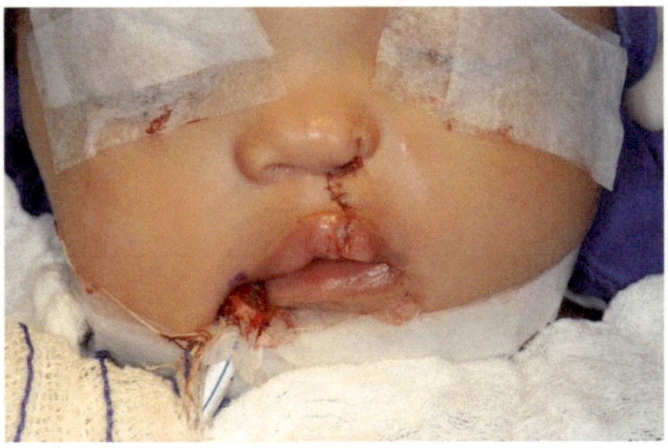

Figure 3.
Primary closure of the labial cleft, in which the reorientation of the Cupid's bow is prioritized to create a harmonic lip. Author: Case report from Oral and Maxillofacial Department of "Defeitos da Face" Medical Center, Sao Paulo, Brazil.

4.2.1 Von Langenbeck technical surgery approach

The Von Lagenbeck technique (in **Figures 4** and 5), described in 1861, is the oldest and used currently. It is usually indicated in the correction of incomplete clefts in order to modify and correct the hard palate. This technique consists of the closure of the palate, from mucoperiosteal flaps, approximated from wide lateral relaxing incisions.

One of the limitations of this technique is the possible occurrence of velopharyngeal insufficiency, consequent to the absence of palatal elongation. Relaxation incisions provide less tension in the tissues and thus lower incidence of oronasal fistulas [18] (**Figures 4** and 5).

4.3 Reconstruction of the alveolar cleft

The alveolar clefts are not treated along with the primary surgeries for correction of the labial and palatal clefts. This is due to the numerous studies published that in the patients who underwent grafts called "primary" grafts in the first years of life, there was a restriction of the transverse growth of the upper maxilla than in

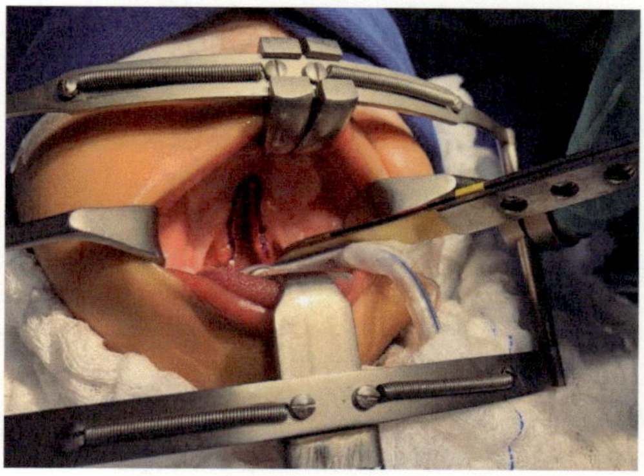

Figure 4.
Post-foraminal complete cleft palate. Author: Case report from Oral and Maxillofacial Department of "Defeitos da Face" Medical Center, Sao Paulo, Brazil.

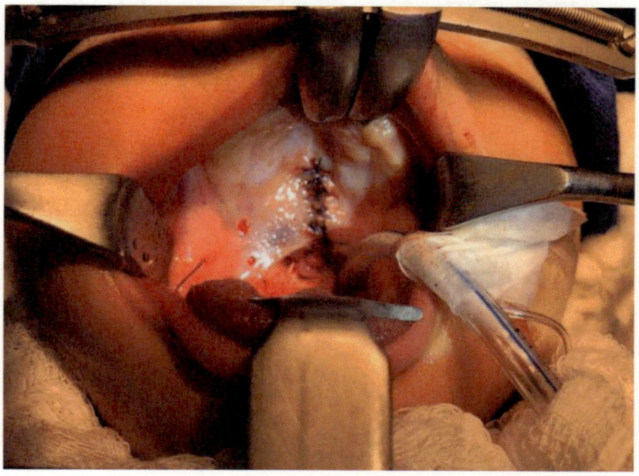

Figure 5.
Primary closure of palate cleft by Von Langenbeck technique surgical approach. Author: Case report from Oral and Maxillofacial Department of "Defeitos da Face" Medical Center, Sao Paulo, Brazil.

the group that was performed in 1 s surgical time, resulting in another long-term surgery to correct this new bone deformity [19–21]. Thus, alveolar reconstruction surgeries remain for another surgical time, where they will be discussed individually.

The advantages of bone grafts in the alveolar clefts are numerous:

1. The existing fistula can be closed between the nasal and oral medium;

2. Possibility of canine eruption in a normal positioning;

3. To help in order to prevent relapse and atresia of the maxillary arch;

4. A bone base is created for the nasal and labial structure, helping to restore not only functionality, but the esthetics of these structures (thus, restorative nasal surgeries should be performed only after alveolar graft surgery).

4.3.1 Phases for the alveolar graft

The alveolar graft is usually performed according to the position of the permanent canine, central incisor, i.e., the permanent incisor tooth must be erupted, and the canine remained in the maxilla or mandibular arch.

The ideal age patient is between 8 and 12 years, as reported in the study by Boyne and Sands [21] (but this age might just be altered due to the eruption position of the canine, referred to chronological age versus dental age).

If a maxillary atresia with a necessity for bone grafting evidenced in alveolar cleft, the maxillary expansion should be performed previously. Moreover, it will facilitate the approach to the alveolar fissure in the graft procedure (**Figure 6**). Not least, once the bone graft has been placed, the expansion will have been become more difficult. Therefore, it would be recommended to perform grafting earlier, even in adult patients.

4.3.2 Surgical technique approach

A mucoperiosteal incision should be performed extending from the ipsilateral side of the alveolar cleft addressed from the height position of three posterior teeth referred to the cleft and up to two teeth later to the midline face.

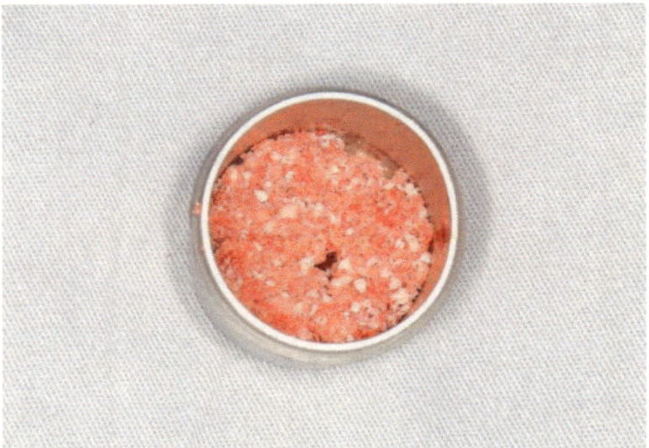

Figure 6.
Particulate autology graft associated with particulate allogeneic (bovine) graft, which is considered the best option for reconstruction of large alveolar fissures. Author: Case report from Oral and Maxillofacial Department of "Defeitos da Face" Medical Center, Sao Paulo, Brazil.

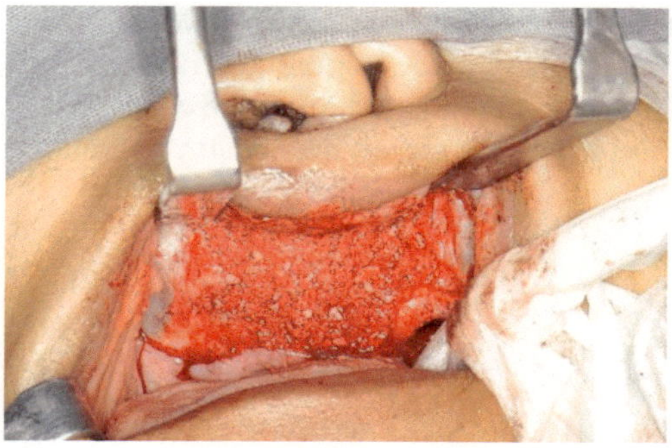

Figure 7.
Adapted particulate graft throughout the cleft region. Author: Case report from Oral and Maxillofacial Department of "Defeitos da Face" Medical Center, Sao Paulo, Brazil.

The aim of this surgical approach, besides the bone graft, is to obtain throughout primary close of all the tissues layers (buccal, nasal, and palatal mucosa) (**Figure 7**).

If this could not occur, the graft might be exposed to the oral cavity and infected. If there will have not been performed an adequate closure of nasal mucosa, it will be possible to create a nasal communication and discharge may occur with as consequence of infection in bone graft.

The management of soft tissue is of great importance in this type of surgical procedure, as well as in the other surgical approaches such as cheiloplasty and palatoplasty.

5. Complications of surgical procedures

The procedures involving the surgical corrections of the lip-palate clefts are extremely delicate surgeries to perform as previously described; however, many corrections are often necessary to achieve desirable results for our patients mainly.

Since primary surgeries, multiple complications may occur from surgical techniques, thus increasing the number of procedures that these patients undergone throughout their lives.

The purpose of next paragraphs will be to discuss the complications of each procedure in the patient with cleft lip and palate.

5.1 Cheiloplasty or plastic surgery lip

Cheiloplasty aims at the correction of the cleft lip. And several techniques are described in the literature for correction (Fisher, Millard, Tennyson-Cronin, among others). However, according to the degree of difficulty of the cleft lip, hypertrophic scars may result as complication of surgery approach, as well as tissue dehiscence and asymmetry between the Cupid's bow treated (cleft) lip and the healthy side.

5.2 Palatoplasty or plastic palate surgery

Palatoplasty has a residual complication such as fistulae on hard and/or soft palate, otitis media, velopharyngeal insufficiency and alteration in maxillofacial growth.

5.3 Secondary/late graft

The grafts are highly exposed to tissue dehiscence in the vestibular region of the alveolar mucosa as well as in the palatal region.

If the primary closure of the three tissue layers would have not been happened during the surgical procedure, it could augmented risk of oronasal communication.

A major one resorption than expected might be observed.

Not least, a secretion in the FO region may occur, and may compromise surgery.

Author details

Henrique Cabrini Moreira[1] and Wilber Bernaola-Paredes[2*]

1 Department of Oral and Maxillofacial Surgery, at Hospital dos Defeitos da Face, São Paulo, Brazil

2 Department of Oral Diagnosis, Oral Medicine and Stomatology at A.C. Camargo Cancer Center, São Paulo, Brazil

*Address all correspondence to: ebernaola@usp.br

References

[1] Aquino SN et al. A review of seasonality of cleft births—The Brazil experience. Journal of Oral Biology and Craniofacial Research. 2017;7(1):2-6

[2] Gkatindis N, Papamanou DA, Christou P, Topouzelis N. Aesthetic outcome of cleft lip and palate treatment. Perceptions of patients, families, and health professionals compared to the general public. Journal of Cranio-Maxillo-Facial Surgery. 2013:e105-e110

[3] Naros A, Brocks A, Kluba S, Reinert S, Krimmel M. Health-related quality of life in cleft lip and/or palate patients—A cross-sectional study from preschool age until adolescence. Journal of Cranio-Maxillo-Facial Surgery. 2018;**46**(10):1758-1763

[4] Klassen AFR, Tsangaris E, Forrest CR, Wong KWY, Pusic AL, Cano SJ, et al. Quality of life of children treated for cleft lip and/or palate: A systemic review. Journal of Plastic, Reconstructive & Aesthetic Surgery. 2012;**65**:547-557

[5] Sharama VP, Bella H, Cadier MM, Pigott RW, Goodacre TEE, Richard BM. Outcomes in facial aesthetics in cleft lip and palate surgery: A systemic review. Journal of Plastic, Reconstructive & Aesthetic Surgery. 2012;**65**:1233-1245

[6] Munz SM, Edwards SP, Inglehart MR. Oral health-related quality of life, and satisfaction with treatment and treatment outcomes of adolescents/young adults with cleft lip/palate: An exploration. International Journal of Oral and Maxillofacial Surgery. 2011;**40**:790-796

[7] Hunt O, Burden D, Hepper P, Johnston C. The psychosocial effects of cleft lip and palate: A systematic review. European Journal of Orthodontics. 2005;**27**:274-285

[8] Popoff DAV, Coelho MP, Martelli DRB, Saini R, Coletta RD. Non-syndromic oral clefts and risk of cancer: A systematic review. Dentistry. 2013;**3000**(1):1-7

[9] Spina V, Psillakis JM, Lapa FS, Ferreira MC. Classificação das fissuras lábio-palatinas: sugestão de modificação. Revista do Hospital das Clínicas da Faculdade de Medicina da Universidade de São Paulo. 1972;**27**(1):5-6

[10] Spina V. A proposed modification for the classification of cleft lip and palate. The Cleft Palate Journal. 1973;**5**(2):251-252

[11] Silva-Filho OG, Ferrari-Júior FM, Rocha DL, Souza-Freitas JA. Classificação das fissuras lábio-palatais: breve histórico, considerações clínicas e sugestão de modificação. Revista Brasileira de Cirurgia. 1992;**82**(2):59-65

[12] Millard DR. Cleft Craft. Vol. 1. Boston (MA): Little Brown; 1976. pp. 165-173

[13] Millard DR. A primary camouflage of the unilateral harelip. In: Transactions of the International Congress of Plastic Surgeons. Baltimore (MD): Williams & Wilkins; 1957. pp. 160-166

[14] La Rossa D. The state of the art in cleft palate surgery. The Cleft Palate-Craniofacial Journal. 2000;**37**(3):225-228

[15] Habel A, Sell D, Mars M. Management of cleft lip and palate. Archives of Disease in Childhood. 1996;**74**:360-366

[16] Agrawal K. Cleft palate repair and variations. Indian Journal of Plastic Surgery. 2009;**42**(Suppl):102-109

[17] Furlow LT Jr. Cleft palate repair by double opposing z-plasty. Plastic and Reconstructive Surgery. 1986;**78**(6):724-738

[18] Eppley B. Alveolar cleft bone grafting (part I): Primary bone grafting. Journal of Oral and Maxillofacial Surgery. 1996;**54**:74-82

[19] Rosenstein SW. Early bone grafting of alveolar cleft deformities. Journal of Oral and Maxillofacial Surgery. 2003;**61**:1078-1081

[20] Brattstrom V, McWilliam J. The influence of bone grafting age on dental abnormalities and alveolar bone height in patients with unilateral cleft lip and palate. European Journal of Orthodontics. 1989;**11**:351-358

[21] Boyne PJ, Sands NR. Combined orthodontics-surgical management of residual palate-alveolar cleft defects. American Journal of Orthodontics. 1976;**70**:20-377

Chapter 3

Deformity of Craniofacial Skeleton by Traumatic Injuries

Raja Kummoona

Abstract

Road traffic crashes on highways with high speed cars can end with termination of life. Immediately after the accident, the medical management includes early transportation by ambulance with highly equipped machines, skilled nurses and doctors to check blood pressure, blood loss, and breathing, administration of intravenous fluid plasma and collecting blood samples for blood grouping. Other treatment can be undertaken by ambulance staff such as temporary splinting (SPICA) of fractured legs and neck support. A helicopter may be used for urgent transport of injured patients with multiple injuries to highly equipped intensive care units in general hospitals. The cooperation of different specialties is required, such as neurosurgeons, craniomaxillofacial surgeons, chest surgeons, general surgeons, and orthopedic surgeons. The order of priority is head injuries, chest injuries, and abdominal injuries. Neglecting early treatment opportunities or delaying treatment results in severe deformities of the facial skeleton and damage to growth of the face in children, leading to severe deformity of the face. Isolated injuries to the eye orbit, nose, jaws, and temporo-mandibular joint (TMJ) may end in ankylosis of the joint in children. A series of clinical cases will be shown.

Keywords: trauma, injuries, craniofacial, deformity

1. Introduction

Road traffic accidents (RTA) in highways occur due to a crash between cars or motorcycles and these crashes cause very common injuries worldwide. It's a disaster and can end in severe injuries to the drivers and passengers. There have been great advances in injury management and in the prevention of these severe cases; some of them with multiple injuries.

There are many steps in the process of early transportation to hospital by ambulance, with highly trained personnel with fully equipped ambulances. The process starts with checking blood pressure, pulse rate, measuring oxygen saturation, giving IV fluid, collecting plasma and blood samples for blood grouping, checking blood sugar. In cases with severe bleeding from the nose and mouth, they have to open the airways by performing a tracheotomy before reaching the emergency room in the hospital. Helicopter transportation might be used for critical cases with multiple injuries such as head injuries, severe facial skeleton injuries, chest injuries, abdominal injuries, and limb injuries [1].

There have been great advances in the radiological diagnostic tools including ultrasound and Doppler, three-dimension CT scan, MRI, and radiological X-ray equipment, including tomography with advances in biochemistry analysis. All these tools assist in the evaluation of the severity of injuries, in addition to proper clinical examination.

Many steps are taken to reduce the severities of car crashes with less damage to the head, chest, and abdominal organs by controlling the rate of speed, preventing alcohol consumption during driving, the wearing of helmet for motorcycle drivers, and compulsory shoulder seatbelts and seat restraints with a special chair for children in the back seat [1].

Vehicle safety measures are incorporated during the manufacturing of cars, from manufacturing air bags to protect the driver and all passengers in small cars, to having safety glass beads with collapsible steering to reduce the trauma to the head, face, and chest. Children should sit in the back in a special seat. All these measures have significantly reduced the incidence of road traffic crashes in both children and adults.

1.1 Materials, results and discussion

As we reported previously in 2011, clinical studies included 673 patients with craniofacial injuries and there were 530 males and 143 females, in the age range between 1 and 75 years (mean 38 years).

Distribution of injuries was as follows: fracture of the mandible 287 (42.64%), middle third injuries 39 (5.79%), and orbital injuries 236 (35.07%) including 12 cases of cranio-orbital ethmoidal injuries. In children, we reported 27 cases (4.0%) of the total cases, we reported also 52 cases that represent (7.73%) zygomatic complex, and zygoma and fracture nose were reported in 40 cases, which form (5.94%) the total cases. 1.

The many advances in the treatment of craniomaxillofacial injuries have been achieved by improvements in medication, tools of diagnosis, and anesthetic machines and medication. These are in addition to the skills and expertise of the anesthetists and care of injured patients by advancing trauma life support by application of the Kummoona 4 golden C rules and ATLAS [2] by,

1. Control of breathing and maintenance of patient airway (tracheotomy sometimes required).

2. Control shock and circulation by intravenous fluid (IV), plasma, and blood after blood grouping.

3. Control of bleeding by cauterization of small vessels and ligation of large vessels.

4. Control of bone fragments and soft tissue laceration.

Craniomaxillofacial injuries have been classified as follows:

A. Craniomaxillofacial injuries with cerebrospinal fluid (CSF) leakage

B. Fractures of middle thirds Le Fort I, Le Fort II, and Le Fort III and sometimes with midline split of the face with or without CSF leakage

C. Fracture of mandible and other isolated injuries such as simple zygoma fracture or more complicated zygomatic complex, orbital skeleton complex and isolated nose fracture.

The most common anatomical area damaged in severe road traffic accidents in the cranial region was the frontal bone with anterior cranial fossa, roof of both orbits, and nose with Dura tears and CSF leakage with head injury [1–3].

The facial skeleton consists of fifty small bones articulating like a pyramid, the top of the pyramid is the nasal tip. Seldom is only one bone of the facial skeleton fractured. The shape and function of the facial skeleton boney articulation acts as a shock absorber and cushion to absorb the impact of trauma and this is because these small bones of the facial skeleton also absorb the force of mastication transmitted along and through the buttress of bones to the base of the skull and this shock absorber of the facial skeleton also protects the vital structures from severe trauma to the underlying vital structures of vision, hearing, smell, taste, speech, and swallowing.

In children, the growth of the face is not completed, except the orbit, in 7 years. Once trauma has occurred, the impact of severe trauma can displace the middle third of the face downward and backward by 45°, with the palate of the maxilla positioned on the dorsum of the tongue, obstructing oral airway with profuse bleeding from fractured nose due to injuries to ethmoidal arteries obstructing nasal airway. This combination of injuries is associated with head injuries, chest injuries, and abdominal injuries and is critical and a life threatening condition.

If children survived from these injuries, they usually recover quickly. Mistreated cases end with severe deformities of the craniofacial region because they received great damage to the growth centers in the cranial sutures, base of skull (sphenoid-occipital synchondrosis), cartilage of the nose, and primary growth center in the condyle.

Treatment of craniomaxillofacial trauma injuries requires expertise, skills and knowledge and these injuries should be treated in highly equipped cranial-maxillofacial centers. Mismanagement or delays in treatment end with severe deformities of the craniofacial region and end by destroying the life of the victim. Even an isolated fracture of the nose, orbit, zygoma, or jaw can end with obvious deformity in a time where people are very concerned about their appearances.

Our aim was directed to prevent complications, deformities, and to restore the normal function and esthetic features of the craniofacial region.

Severe cases of craniomaxillofacial injuries with head injuries and chest injuries need to be admitted immediately to an intensive care unit for a few days until the patient has recovered from the head and chest injuries before adequate treatment of the craniofacial injuries [1–4].

The treatment of a CSF leak usually follows the conservative principle of reduction and repair of craniofacial fractures through the following steps:

1. Reduction of intra cranial pressure (ICP) by elevation of the head by 45°

2. Reduction of CSF leakage using carbonic anhydrase inhibitors (Acetazolamide {Diamox 3-kcl})250 mg twice daily, to correct hyperkalemia as a complication of Diamox and 4 triple antibiotics to prevent meningitis

3. The CSF leak usually stops within 4–5 days. If the CSF does not stop, a lumber puncture is required to reduce the ICP by aspiration of CSF

4. If the CSF leakage does not stop after all the previous procedures and measurement, perform a craniotomy indicated for Dura repair by piece of Gale aponeurosis or a piece of temporalis muscle and sutured watertight.

The treatment of head injuries is the responsibility of the neurosurgeon, with collaboration of the craniofacial surgeon [2].

We undertook research on CSF analysis by taking several samples from patients with head injuries and blood serum from the same patients to study the differences between the two samples. We used a high specific isoelectric focusing electrophoresis set on polyacrylamide gel for direct immunofixation of transferrin by a plex electrophoresis set and spectrophotometer for serum sample. Using this study, we can detect the CSF leakage due to traumatic injuries and differentiate it from serum exudate.

Through this research we were able to detect the concentration of the B2-Transferrin enzyme in CSF and this level was 90.26 ppm, which represents about 35 times more than that detected in serum exudate [1].

The facial skeleton and the face are the mirror of the body reflecting happiness, sadness, beauty, and ugliness. The face is a mirror of intelligence and dullness and it also shows the body's signs of disease such as paleness, dryness of skin, yellow skin, dark or bluish skin, blisters, or pigments. These are all features of illness.

2. Clinical features, deformities and treatments

Trauma to the face and subsequent deformities is a disaster to the patient and our duty is to restore the normal architecture of the face by restoring esthetic and functional activity of the facial skeleton. The problem is that the face is not padded by clothing and traumatic impact has a direct effect on the soft and hard tissue of the face. Once an accident has happened, we have to direct our effort to repair the soft tissue properly as the first step and to put every piece of bone of the facial skeleton in its anatomical position and to fix it either by plating or by soft stainless steel wires of 0.25 and 0.5 mm as a basic principle. Soft tissue damage may be a laceration or loss of soft tissue and these are repaired using local rotational flaps or regional flaps such as the forehead flap or Kummoona lateral cervical flap [5].

Deformities of the frontal bone and anterior cranial fossa can occur with severe trauma to the area associated with severe nasal-ethmoidal-orbital bone injuries with CSF leakage and head injuries. Serious injuries require admission to intensive care units until the patient recovers from the head injuries. A craniotomy through a bi-coronal flap is used for exploration of the anterior cranial fossa after retraction of the brain. Dura are repaired by galea aponeurosis or a piece of temporalis muscle with watertight suturing with silk and reconstruction of the anterior cranial fossa and the roofs of both orbits by bone grafting from the iliac crest. The frontal bone is repaired by bone graft or by rubber silicone material (Sialastic). The nose can be reduced at the same time [3] (**Figures 1–3**).

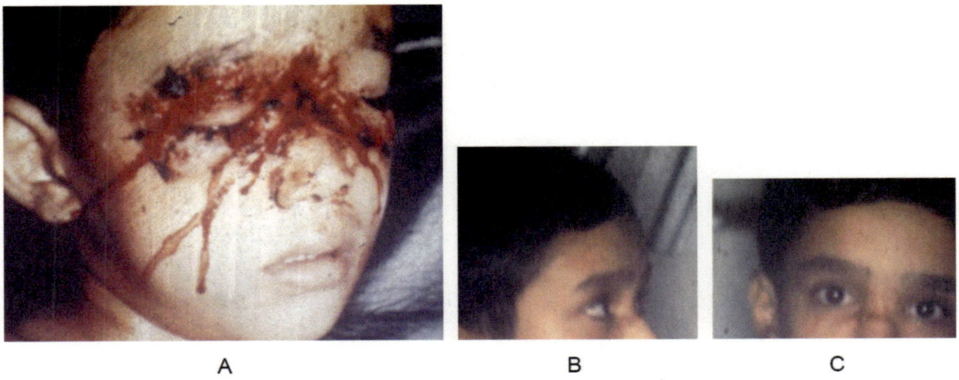

Figure 1.
(A) Severe traumatic injuries to the nasal-ethmoidal-orbital region with laceration of overlying skin in a 4-year-old boy. (B and C) Post-operative photo after reconstruction of the region after 2 years.

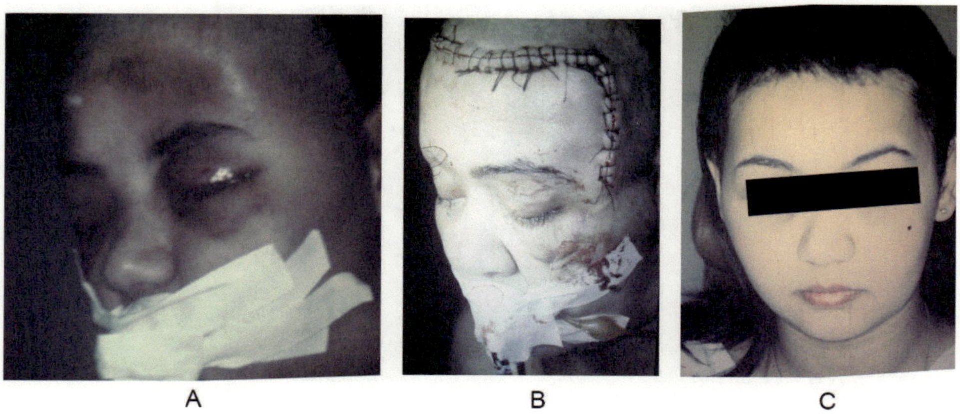

Figure 2.
(A) Severe road traffic accident with deformity of cranial-facial region with damage to frontal bone, anterior cranial fossa with Dura tear, CSF leakage, and nasal-ethmoidal-orbital skeleton and nasal bone. (B) Bi-coronal flap used for craniotomy and for exploration of the anterior cranial fossa, for reconstruction of Dura, anterior cranial fossa, roof of the orbits, frontal bone, and nasal-ethmoidal-orbital region by bone graft and Sialastic implant. (C) Post-operative photo after 3 months showing slight dislocation of medial canthal ligament.

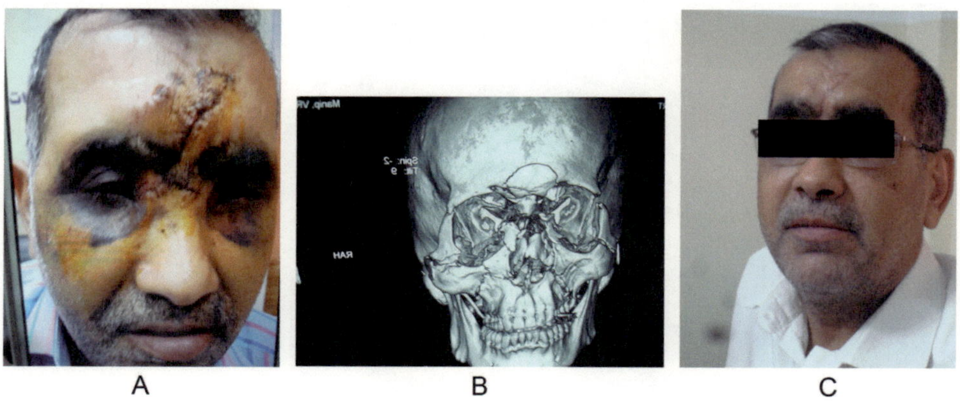

Figure 3.
(A) Severe injuries from a road traffic accident to the craniofacial region with CSF leakage, elongation of the face, and displacement of the facial skeleton downward and backward. (B) 3D CT scan of the face showing the severity of the injuries. (C) Three months post-operative photo showing restoration of the facial skeleton after several operations.

Deformities of the face can occur either to the whole facial skeleton in a scattered manner or to a part of it, such as the orbital skeleton damage with the globe of the eyes, an isolated fracture roof with downward displacement of eye ball, a fracture of the medial wall with dislocation of medial canthi and damage to nasolacrimal duct with enophthalmos, fracture of the floor of the orbit featuring diplopia and enophthalmos, or fracture of the zygoma and lateral wall with displacement of the zygomatic bone either downward or laterally or rotated or inward.

In more severe cases with compression of the superior orbital fissures, this can result in superior orbital fissure syndrome and will be manifested as exophthalmos, ptosis, ophthalmoplegia, and fixed pupil with loss of vision and loss of sensation in the surrounding area and edema of the eyelids. Immediate treatment may restore the function of the eye and vision by reduction of zygomatic bone and elevation of compression on the superior orbital fissure. If there has been a severe impact with a sharp object to the globe of the eye with severe laceration and with no response of the pupil to light, evisceration of the eye must be performed by an ophthalmologist [6–8] (**Figures 4–6**).

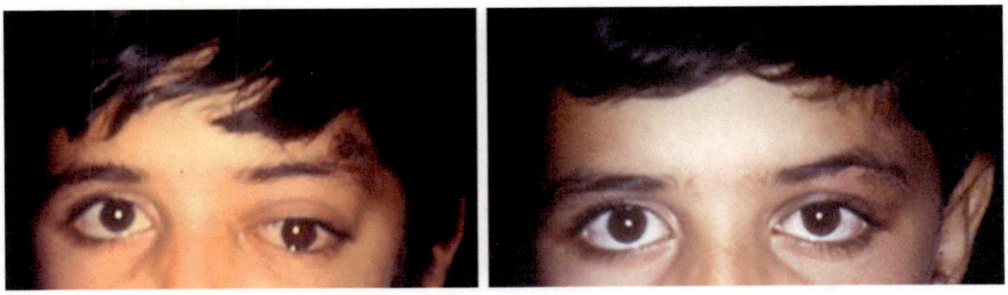

Figure 4.
(A) Deformity of the orbit due to traumatic injuries with downward displaced eyeball due to fracture in the roof of the orbit of a 4-year-old boy. (B) Post-operative photo after reconstruction of the roof of the orbit by Sialastic implant.

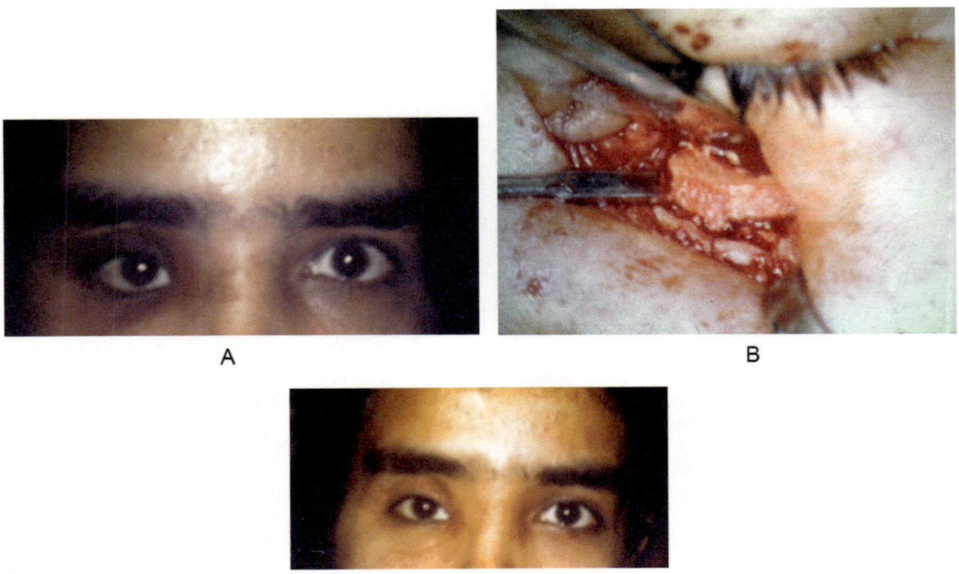

Figure 5.
(A) Severe enophthalmos due to traumatic injury to the floor and medial wall of the orbit with dislocation of medial canthal ligament. (B) Reconstruction of the orbital floor by bone graft from iliac crest. (C) Post-operative photo after reconstruction of the floor and medial wall and fixation of median canthal ligament.

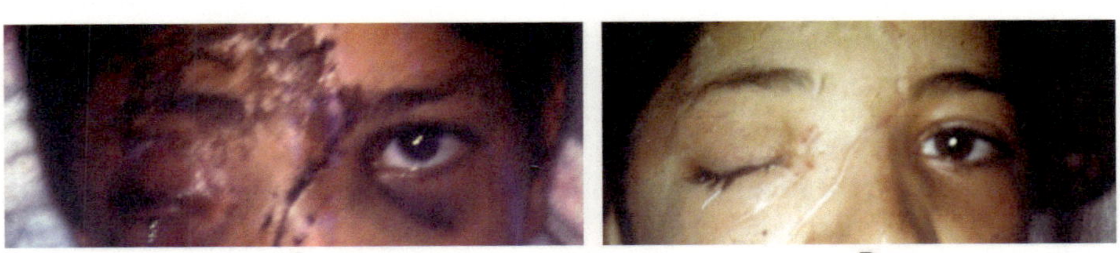

Figure 6.
(A) Severe injuries to orbital skeleton and content with loss of eyeball. (B) Reconstruction of all orbital skeleton with ptosis of upper lid required in a secondary surgery and artificial eyeball.

Bad injuries to the mandible with multiple fractures and delayed treatment can cause severe deformity with open bite and malocclusion. Usually the injuries affect the body and angle either as a favorite fracture or an unfavored fracture. The favorite fracture is not affected by muscles of mastication. The direction of the fracture line plays an important role in preventing displacement. The unfavorite type of fractures of the angle with displacement were affected by temporalis, medial pterygoid, and masseter muscles. These fractures required an open reduction through a submandibular incision, fixation of fragments done by plating or by soft stainless steel wire of 0.5 mm as a double eight crossing each other with inter maxillary fixation (IMF). A less severe form of this fracture angle might be treated by upper border wiring with IMF (**Figure 7A–D**).

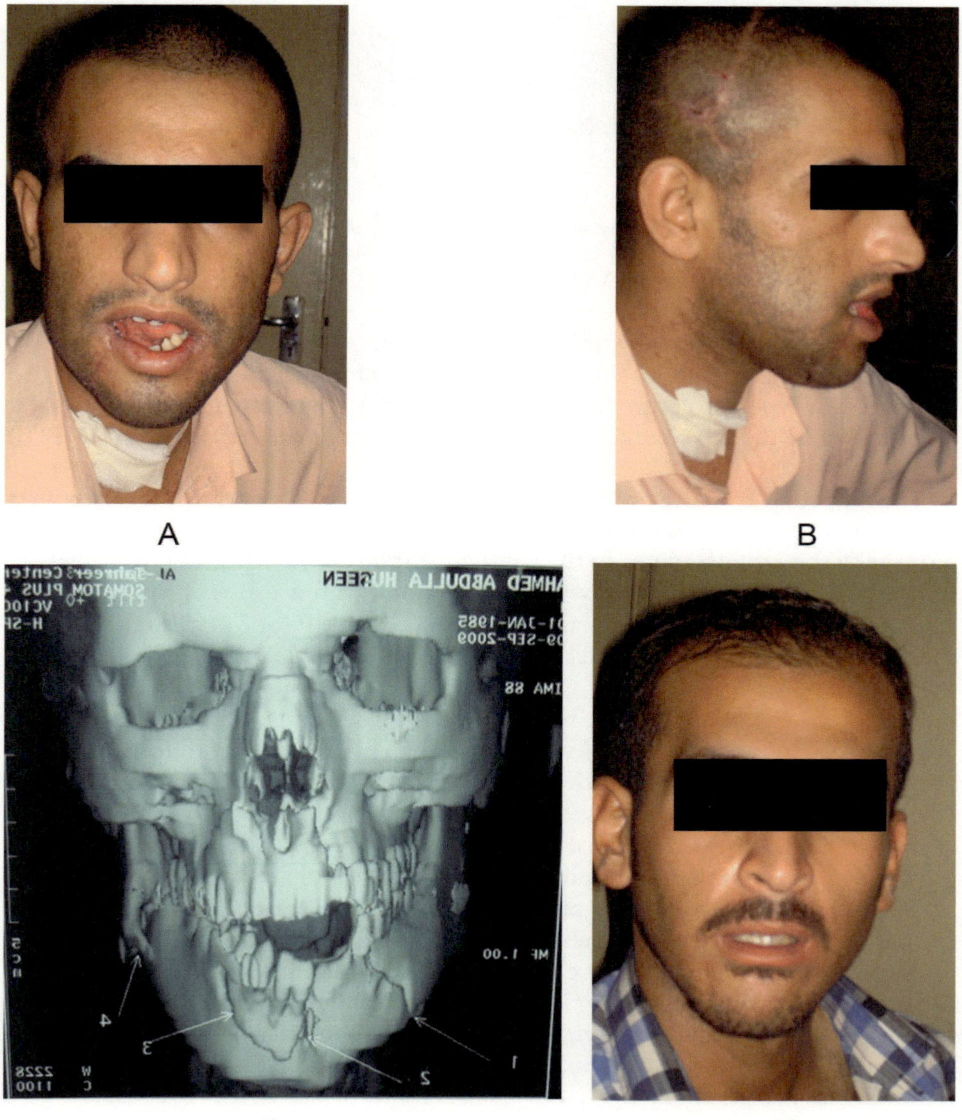

Figure 7.
(A and B) Severe traumatic deformity of the mandible with open bite and injuries to cranial region with head injury and CSF leakage treated by craniotomy and Dural repair. (C) 3D CT scan of lower jaw showing multiple injuries. (D) Six months post-operative photo.

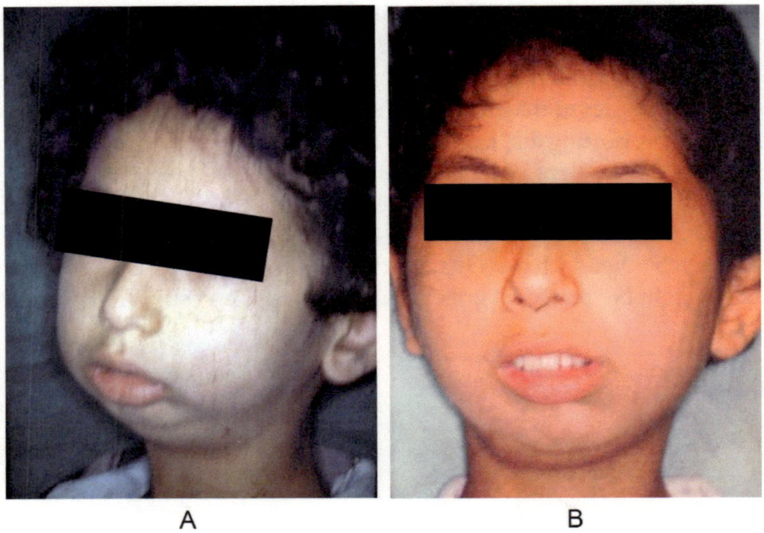

Figure 8.
(A) Severe deformity of the mandible due to intra-uterine injuries to the right temporo-mandibular joint and the child born with ankylosis of the TMJ. (B) One year post-operative after reconstruction of the right TMJ by Kummoona Chonro-Ossous graft at age of 5 years.

The other types of fracture affect the ramus and the most common two types of fractures are the condylar (intra capsular) type and sub condylar type. The intracapsular type of fracture condyle is a very serious injury that requires special attention while the sub condylar type is treated by inter maxillary fixation (IMF) for 3–4 weeks.

Intracapsular fracture of the condyle in children is very serious. If mistreated, it can lead to ankylosis with severe deformity of the mandible and midface due to damage to the growth center in the condyle. Early treatment of an intracapsular fracture should be carried out by administration of a few drops of hydrocortisone to prevent adhesion and to reduce edema with IMF for 3–4 days to relief spasm of muscles and to remodel the shape of the condyle followed by early mobilization.

Once adhesion of the condyle had occurred and deformity of the jaw has appeared, we must excise the ankylosed joint with hyperplastic coronoid, re-attach of the muscles of mastication and reconstruct the TMJ by using Kummoona Chondro-Osseous graft was harvested from iliac crest in children for restoration of growth, remodeling, and repair of the condyle (**Figure 8**). The graft can restore the growth of the mandible and midface and prevent residual deformity [2, 4, 6]..

In craniofacial injuries, after reconstruction of the anterior cranial fossa and frontal bone, we have immediately to reduce and fix the middle third fracture of the facial skeleton including Le Fort I, II, III, and mid line split of the face. Reduction was achieved by using Rowe dis impaction forceps to move the displaced facial skeleton upward and forward in the reverse direction of the displacement of the middle third and to put the skeleton in its normal anatomical position with intermaxillary fixation (IMF).

Fixation of the facial skeleton was performed by using our techniques of fixation by suspension of middle third through the sandwich technique using soft stainless steel wire of 0.5 mm and making hole by using round bur in the frontal-zygomatic suture above the fracture line and the wire is passed below the zygoma down through the cheek to the lower arch bar fixed by wires and IMF and reinforced by a circum-mandibular wire with proper occlusion of the teeth.

Another technique is the Halo Frame fixed by 4 pins to the skull and again two cheek wires attached to the Halo Frame and passed below the zygoma to the upper or lower arch bar. Another technique is the Box frame technique that requires insertion of 4 pins (2 in the frontal process of the frontal bone and 2 pins in the angle of the lower jaw) with 4 rods fixed after reduction of the displaced midface with IMF to achieve proper occlusion. The success of treatment is based on proper occlusion and proper fixation of the small bones of the facial skeleton to be sited in their anatomical position and to get normal facial length and height.

3. Conclusion

The aim of our research is to share our techniques and expertise in the treatment and management of traumatic craniofacial deformities with other colleagues worldwide.

In this clinical research, we studied 673 patients with craniofacial injuries and deformities and the incidence of these injuries to affect various parts of craniofacial region, we did classify these injuries and how serious ,primary care described thoroughly and cases with cranial or LeFort III injuries might associated with CSF leakage ,methods of management were described by conservative technique if not by craniotomy. Different techniques for reduction and fixation of the craniofacial regions were also described.

This study shows the ability of the author to deal with very difficult cases of craniofacial region. I hope this chapter satisfies the curiosity of the readers.

Author details

Raja Kummoona
Council of Maxillofacial Surgery, Iraqi Board for Medical Specialization, Baghdad, Iraq

*Address all correspondence to: raja_kummoona@hotmail.com

References

[1] Kummoona R. Managements of maxillofacial injuries in Iraq. Journal of Craniofacial Surgery. 2011;**22**:1561-1567

[2] Kummoona R. Pediatrics maxillofacial injuries with special attention to fracture condyle. EC Pediatrics. 2017;**5**(6):170-171

[3] Kummoona R. Orbital trauma with special references to pediatrics and chilidren. EC Pediatrics. 2018;**7**(5)

[4] Kummoona R. Pediatrics and children facial deformity with special reference to Ankylosis of the TMJ. EC Pediatrics. 2018;**7**(3):112-115

[5] Kummoona R. Kummoona lateral cervical flap for reconstruction of oral defect after cancer surgery. Clinical Case Reports. 2018;**1**(1):1006

[6] Kummoona R. Temporomandibular joint ankylosis that affect children and reconstruction by Kummoona Chondro-Osseous Graft. EC Pediatrics. 2018;**7**(11)

[7] Kummoona R. Pediatrics and chilidren facial deformity with special reference to ankylosis of the temporomandibular joint. EC Pediatrics. 2018;**7**(3):112-115

[8] Kummoona R. Kummoona Chondro-Ossous graft good substitute to condylar growth center and fore correction of facial deformity in children. Archives of Otolaryngology and Rhinology. 2017;**3**(3):098-102

Chapter 4

The Basics of Splinting in Dentoalveolar Traumatology

Naida Hadziabdic

Abstract

Dentoalveolar trauma is considered an emergency condition and is challenging for every dentist. As primary and permanent teeth may suffer repercussions from an injury, a therapist must be mindful of which situations the use of splinting methods is required. In dentistry, a splint is a rigid or flexible device with the function of supporting, protecting, and immobilizing teeth that have been weakened (endodontically, periodontally), traumatically injured, replanted, or fractured. Generally, splinting is not recommended for primary teeth injuries such as luxation and avulsion. In permanent dentition, splint appliances are indicated for periodontal injuries, such as subluxation, luxation and avulsion, and hard tissue injuries such as class IV root fractures. Nowadays, there are many appliances that may be used for immobilization of traumatized teeth. Since this issue may sometimes be confusing for dental practitioners, this chapter deals with splint classification (rigid and flexible), the basic characteristics of splints, the indications, and methods of application.

Keywords: splinting, traumatized teeth, dentoalveolar trauma, immobilization

1. Introduction

Since any dentoalveolar trauma is an emergency condition, it is a challenge for all dentists. Since both primary and permanent teeth may suffer injury, a dental therapist must first of all know the situations in which the use of a splint is indicated as a means of immobilization [1–4].

However, first of all, let us look at what a splint is.

A splint is a rigid or flexible device/aid used to support, protect, and immobilize teeth that have been weakened (endodontically or periodontally), traumatized, replanted, or fractured [5–7].

In order to even consider the use of a splint, it is necessary to know whether the traumatized tooth is primary or permanent and what kind of injury it has suffered.

In general, the use of a splint is not recommended for injuries to milk teeth, such as luxation or avulsion. Luxated milk teeth are most often extracted. Repositioning is not recommended because there is a risk of infection which could endanger the tooth bud of the permanent tooth. An avulsed milk tooth is not replanted [4, 8, 9].

In permanent dentition, the use of a splint is indicated for [10]:

- Injuries to the periodontal tissue (subluxation, luxation, and avulsion)
- Injuries to the hard dental tissue (class IV root fractures)

2. Types of splint

Splints are categorized as:

- Rigid splints
- Nonrigid/semirigid/flexible splints

This categorization of splints is based on the possibility of the physiological mobility of the tooth [11]. Thus, a rigid splint does not permit any physiological mobility of the tooth and thereby creates the conditions for complications in the sense of ankylosis or external resorption [5].

In the case of a nonrigid or semirigid splint, the physiological functional mobility of the traumatized tooth is possible, which is more favorable for the healing of the periodontal ligament (PDL), and thereby the risk of ankylosis or external resorption of the tooth root is reduced [12].

2.1 Types of rigid and semirigid splints

Rigid splints:

- Suture splints
- Arch bar splints
- Acrylic splints
- Composite splints

Semirigid splints:

- Orthodontic brackets and arches
- Wire and composite splints
- Fiber splints
- Titanium trauma splints (TTS)

2.1.1 Rigid splints

2.1.1.1 Suture splints

Soft wire and surgical thread can be used as materials for this type of splint [13–15]. The use of soft wire is indicated for mixed dentition. The wire is woven around the traumatized and neighboring teeth (**Figure 1**). Immobilization of this kind should be brief—only a few days. The weaknesses of this type of immobilization are that the metal thins and breaks with chewing, and it also prevents good oral hygiene, which leads to gingivitis [16].

When there are no neighboring teeth to which the splint may be fixed, the use of a surgical suture is indicated for the sake of immobilization (**Figure 2**).

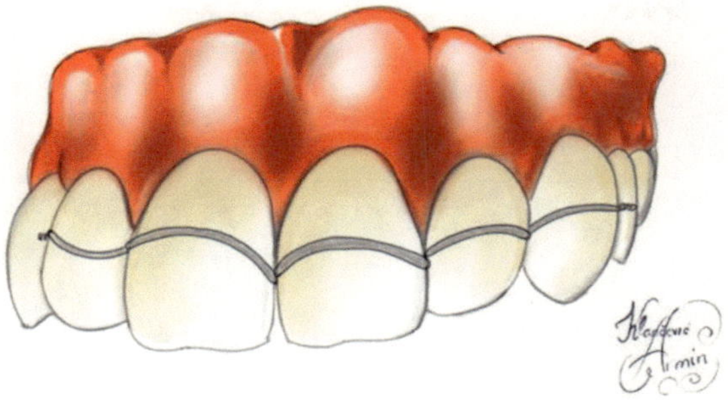

Figure 1.
Wire acting as a suture splint.

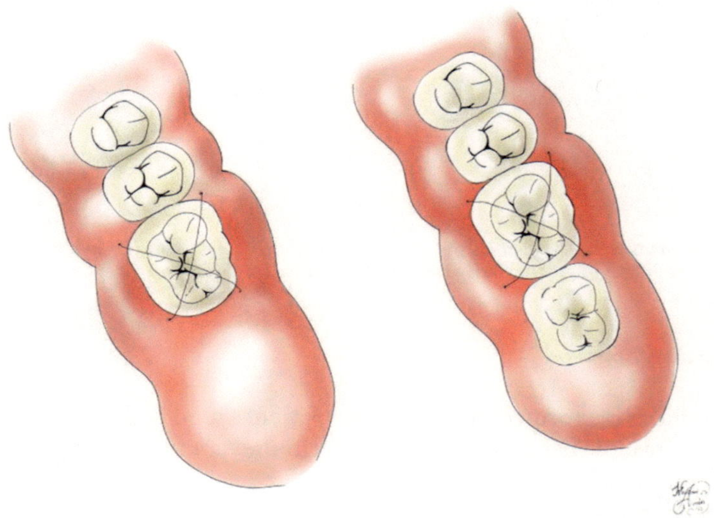

Figure 2.
A surgical suture used as a suture splint.

2.1.1.2 Arch bar splints

These are ready-made metal bars with hooks onto which the wire is woven which fixes the metal brackets to the teeth [17] (**Figure 3**). The bars are placed right up against the gums which cause irritation, and they are therefore impractical for everyday use [18].

2.1.1.3 Acrylic splints

As their name suggests, these splints are made from acrylic material [19, 20]. They are not used for isolated dental traumas. They are indicated in cases of luxation of a tooth in combination with a fracture of the alveolar bone. The best-known splint of this type is the Pfeiffer splint.

This splint may be made in two ways:

- The direct method
- The indirect method

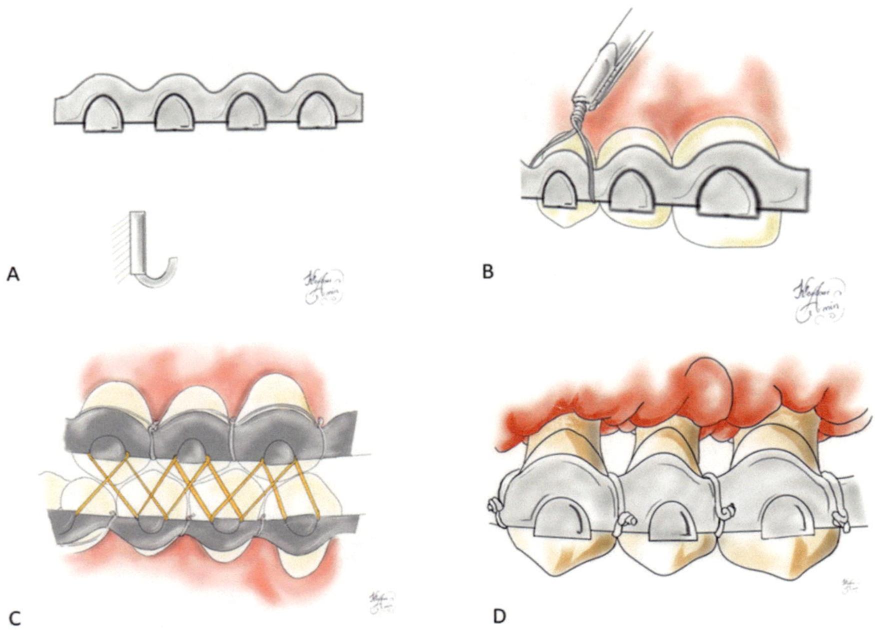

Figure 3.
(A) Ready-made metal arch, (B) metal arch fixed with wire to the upper teeth, (C) intermaxillary fixation, and (D) the appearance of gums after being irritated from the use of a ready-made splint.

2.1.1.3.1 The direct method

This method is performed directly in the patient's mouth, and for that reason, it is very uncomfortable because the acrylic sets in the mouth, creating an unpleasant warm reaction.

The following materials are needed for this method (**Figure 4**):

- Vaseline
- Self-adhesive acrylic (powder and liquid)
- A container for mixing the acrylic
- A piece of sterile gauze
- Glass for mixing
- A spatula for mixing
- Scissors
- Pliers
- Grinder

The procedure (**Figure 5**):

DOI: http://dx.doi.org/10.5772/intechopen.88061

- First of all, establish the type of injury and decide if using a Pfeiffer splint is indicated.
- Check the position of the teeth in central occlusion and remember those positions.
- Blend the acrylic.
- Pour the blended acrylic onto the piece of sterile gauze.
- Use the scissors to cut the edge of the gauze to create a rectangular shape, so the future splint will cover two neighboring teeth on each side of the injured tooth.
- Protect the gums with Vaseline.
- Shape the splint over the vestibular and palatal surfaces of the tooth, tell the patient to bite down, and check the occlusion.
- Once it has set, remove the splint from the mouth.
- Use the grinder on the internal side of the splint to make room for the phosphate cement. In addition, it is necessary to use the grinder to work on the vestibular part of the splint so the cervical third of the crown is exposed, which will make it possible to test the vitality of the tooth while the splint is in place.
- The blended phosphate cement is poured into the prepared splint after which the splint is cemented in the patient's mouth, with verification of the central occlusion.

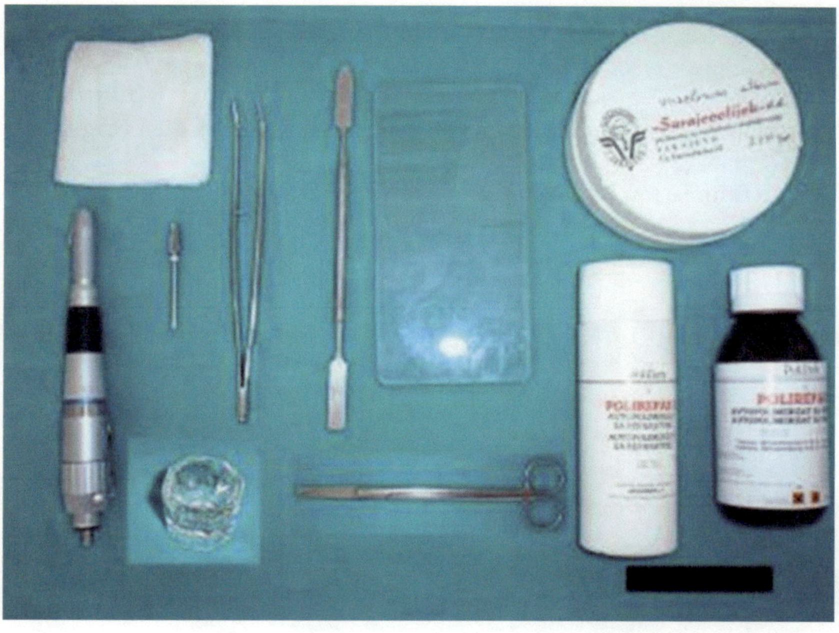

Figure 4.
Equipment for creating an acrylic Pfeiffer splint.

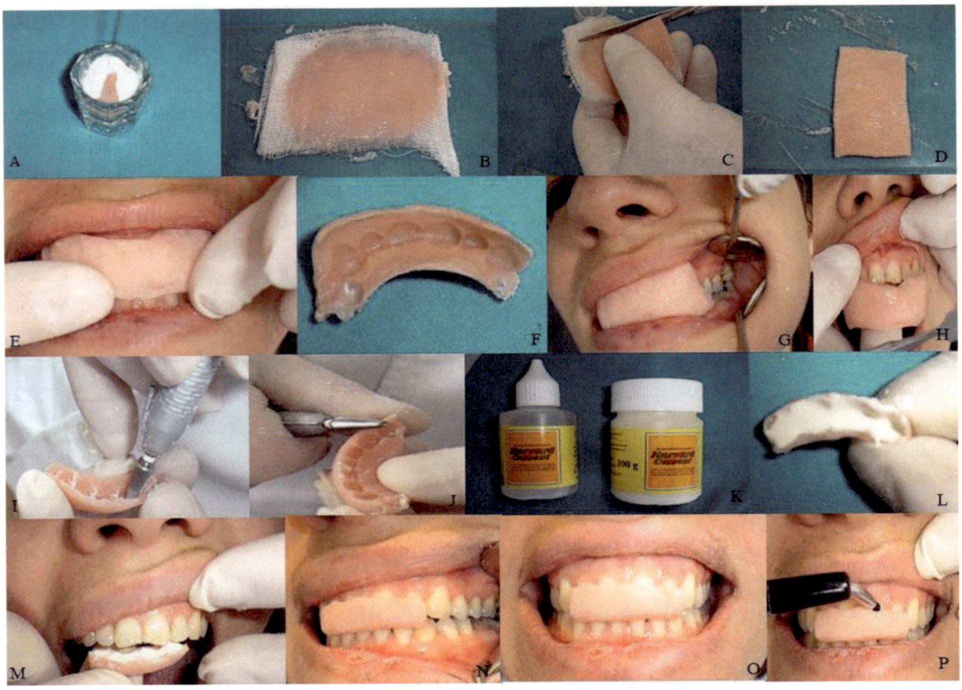

Figure 5.
Creating a Pfeiffer splint using the direct technique: (A) blending the acrylic, (B) pouring the blended acrylic onto the sterile gauze, (C) cutting the edges of the gauze onto which the acrylic was poured, (D) the rectangular-shaped gauze, (E) adjusting the splint over the vestibular and palatal surface of the tooth, (F) the inside of the splint, (G) verification of the splint in central occlusion, (H) removing the splint for processing, (I) creating space for the cement, (J) processing-cutting the edges of the splint, (K) phosphate cement, (L) the final appearance of the splint with the cement inside, (M) cementing the splint, (N) inserting the splint with verification of the central occlusion (side view), (O) the centered splint in the mouth (front view), and (P) testing the vitality of the tooth.

2.1.1.3.2 The indirect method

This method differs from the previous one in how it is executed (**Figure 6**):

- First an impression is taken of the jaw in alginate.
- Various models are created in the laboratory.

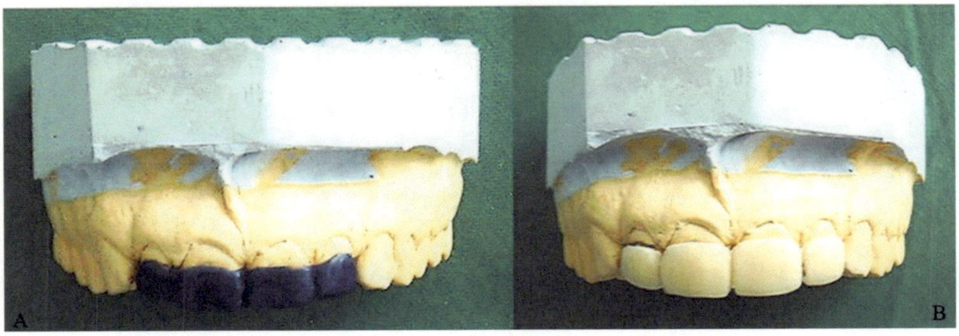

Figure 6.
The indirect method of creating a Pfeiffer splint: (A) the wax model and (B) the acrylic splint on the model.

- On the basis of the models, a splint is created in wax so that the cervical part of the crown of the tooth remains uncovered.
- The wax model is exchanged for acrylic.
- The splint is cemented in the same way as in the previous method.

2.1.1.4 Composite splints

Only composite materials are used to make this kind of splint (**Figure 7**). The technique is very simple because it consists of working with composite material in the classical way:

- Conditioning of the enamel of the injured and neighboring teeth
- Application of the adhesive and composite material with polymerization

The weakness of a composite splint is its tendency to split due to the action of interdental occlusal forces. It also may irritate the surrounding gums if it is placed very close to them.

A so-called interapproximal composite splint is a sub-type of this splint. The specific feature of this splint is that composite material is also placed on the approximal surface of the traumatized and neighboring teeth. This kind of splint is quite insecure and may only be used in cases when there has not been any major damage caused by avulsion and when the neighboring teeth are intact.

2.1.2 Semirigid splints

2.1.2.1 Orthodontic splints

For this type of splint, orthodontic brackets and orthodontic wire are needed [21] (**Figure 8**). The brackets are placed in the middle third of the labial surface of the tooth. They are connected by orthodontic wire, 0.016 mm in diameter, which is passively adapted. There are some who claim that orthodontic wire is not "passive" and that the action of orthodontic forces is possible.

The advantage of immobilization using an orthodontic splint is the possibility of synchronizing the movement of the teeth, which is particularly important in cases of intrusion. The weakness is the irritation of the lips, which can be avoided by applying wax.

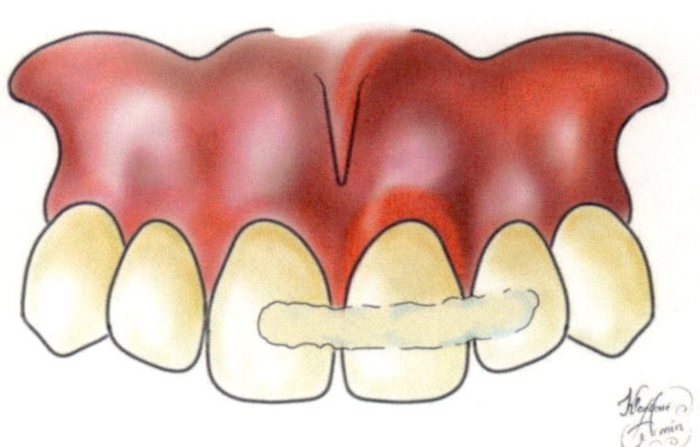

Figure 7.
A splint made exclusively from composite material.

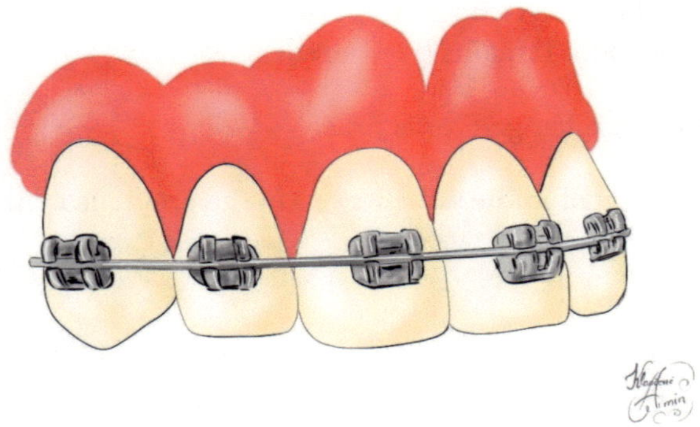

Figure 8.
An orthodontic splint.

2.1.2.2 Wire-composite splints

The splint that is used most often in everyday practice is a wire-composite splint [6, 22]. To make it, any composite material and orthodontic wire, 0.3–0.4 mm in diameter, are needed. It is indicated in all cases of traumatic injuries (**Figure 9**). Contraindications for the use of a wire and composite splint are when the teeth have artificial crowns and large fillings or in the teeth with exceptionally small crowns.

The technique for making one is quite simple:

- Orthodontic wire of the selected length is shaped directly in the patient's mouth to cover 2–3 teeth on each side of the injured tooth.

- The labial surface is conditioned using orthophosphoric acid.

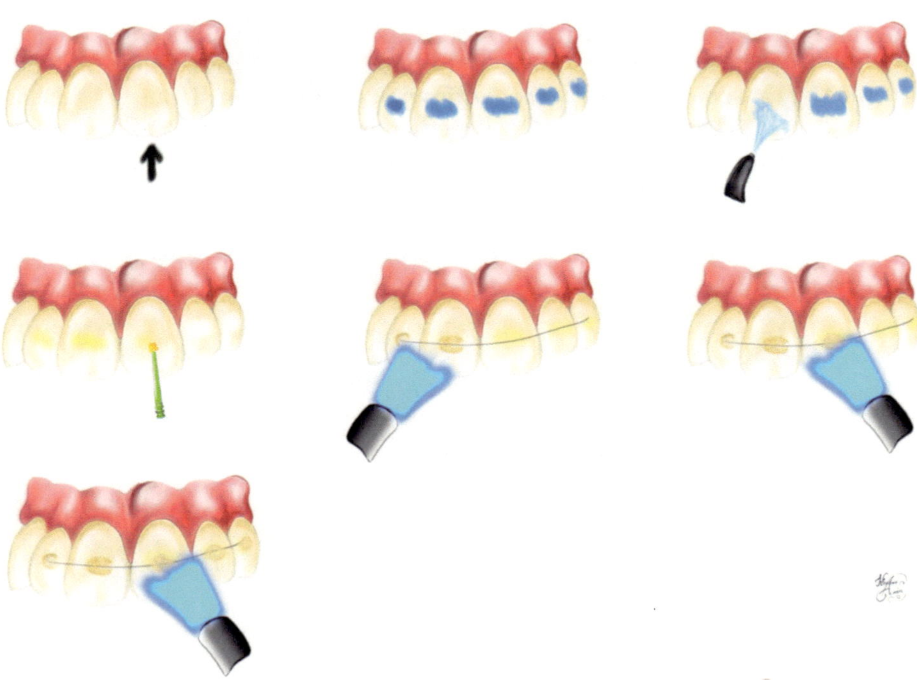

Figure 9.
Making a wire-composite splint.

- After rinsing and drying, they are coated with the bonding substance and light cured for about 10 s.
- The composite material is placed over the tooth and over that an arch, braces, or wire are positioned.
- Light curing should first be performed on the healthy teeth on one side; then the tooth should be repositioned, followed by light curing (polymerization); and then the wire should be light cured on the healthy teeth on the other side.
- In order to avoid shifting a replanted tooth while polymerizing the wires, the splint may also be fixed as follows: after repositioning, the patient bites down on softened wax (as when taking an impression for prosthetics-bite registration). The tooth remains in the desired position during the fixation of the splint to the tooth.

2.1.2.3 Fiber splints

These types of splint include [6, 23, 24]:

- Fishing line [25] (**Figure 10**)
- Glass-ionomer fiber
- Ribbond splint
- Kevlar fiber

Fishing line and glass-ionomer fiber are used in the same way as in a wire-composite splint.

2.1.2.3.1 Ribbond splint

This type of splint relies on the use of special polyethylene fibers, Ribbond fibers, and composite materials [6, 26] (**Figure 11**). In dental traumatology, Ribbond fiber splints are fixed and extra-coronary. They are used intracoronarily in cases of periodontitis, where it is necessary to create cavities in the teeth to place the fiber.

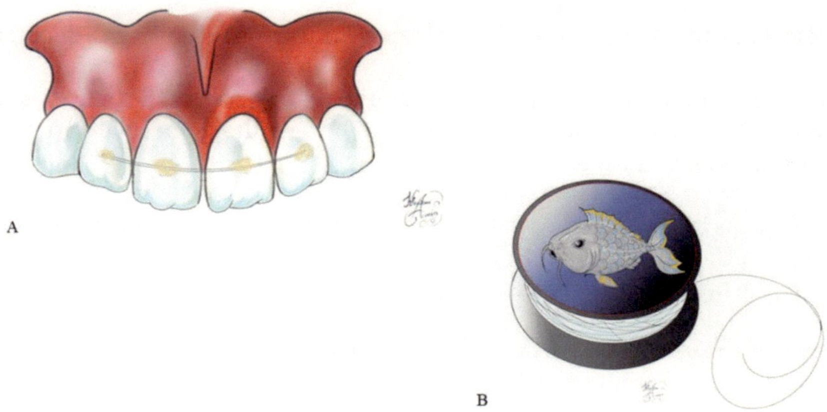

Figure 10.
(A) Fishing line used as a splint and (B) fishing line.

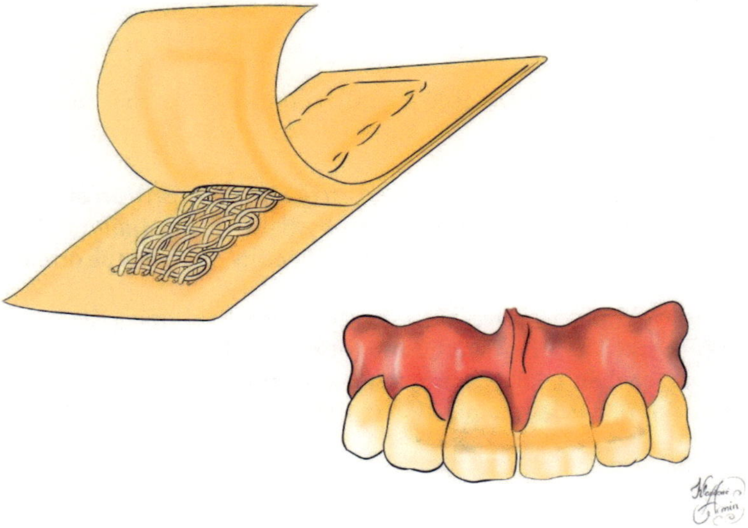

Figure 11.
A Ribbond splint.

Ribbond fibers are popular as a form of immobilization due to their properties:

- They are exceptionally strong, thanks to the special way they are woven.
- The surface of the fiber is treated using an electrochemical plasma procedure, so the mechanical properties of the fibers are improved, as well as bonding to the composite resin.
- Their permeability to light makes work possible with any form of composite material.
- They have excellent properties relating to manipulation.

The technique for placing a Ribbond splint:

- Clean the vestibular surface of the tooth.
- Determine the length of the Ribbond tape (measure the length with dental floss).
- Cut the Ribbond tape using special scissors. In this process the tape must not be touched by hand to avoid contamination. The tape should be held with tweezers or cotton gloves until it is impregnated.
- The tape is impregnated with bonding agent or fissure sealant material.
- Store the tape in a dark place.
- Parts of the vestibular surfaces of the injured and neighboring teeth are conditioned with orthophosphoric acid for 30 s.
- Wash the acid off with water, and dry.

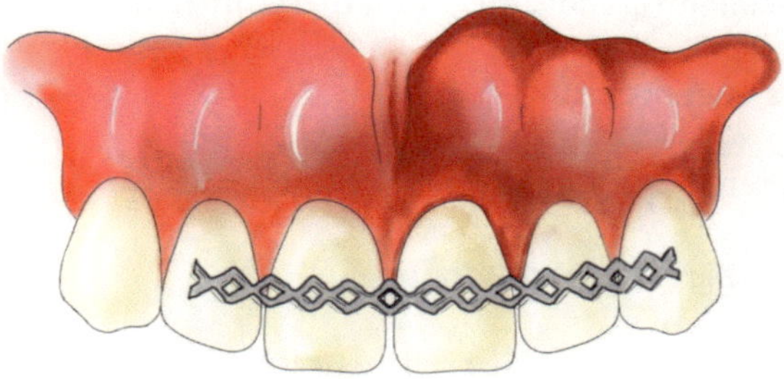

Figure 12.
Titanium trauma splint (TTS).

- Apply the adhesive on the conditioned surface of the teeth.
- Apply the flowable composite material to the tooth and then the Ribbond tape, which is pressed into the composite applied and smoothed, and excess composite material is removed. Each tooth is then light cured for 30–40 s.
- Using a drill, we remove the excess composite material and polish the surface of the composite.

2.1.2.3.2 Kevlar fiber

Kevlar fiber, poly-paraphenylene terephthalamide, is a synthetic, organic fiber of exceptional strength (five times stronger than metal). As well as being used to make bulletproof vests and in the aero-industry, it is used in dental traumatology as a means of immobilizing teeth [6]. It has the identical features, therapeutic effect, and manner of application as Ribbond splints.

2.1.2.4 Titanium trauma splint (TTS)

A TTS is a more recent splint, made from pure titanium, only 0.2 mm in thickness, which makes it significantly easier to apply to the tooth [6, 23, 27–29]. It is available in 52 and 100 mm lengths. It is designed in the form of a rhomboid mesh, which makes it easier to be fixed and makes it flexible in all dimensions (**Figure 12**). The size of the rhomboid opening, 1.8 × 2.8 mm, reduces the quantity of composite material used to fix it to the surface of the tooth, making it easier to remove the splint. It is fixed to the tooth in the same way as a wire-composite splint. The weakness of this splint system is that it is very expensive in comparison with a wire-composite splint.

3. The features of an acceptable splint

In view of the diversity of splints which may be used for traumatized teeth, the following features of a good splint should be used as guidelines in selection [4]:

- It is simple to create and put in place.
- It prevents further traumatization of the injured tooth.

- It enables physiological movement and therefore healing.
- It does not obstruct occlusion.
- It makes maintenance of oral hygiene possible.
- It makes it possible to monitor vitality.
- It does not obstruct endodontic treatment when necessary.
- It is aesthetic.
- It is easily removed.

4. Recommendations for the type and duration of immobilization depending on the type of trauma

In dentoalveolar traumatology, answers have not been found for all the questions that arise, especially regarding the duration of the use of splints. The effect of the duration of immobilization, that is, keeping a splint in place during the healing of the periodontal ligament, has still not been explained in clinical studies. The long-term use of a splint leads to ankylosis and replacement resorption. On the other hand, it has not been confirmed that there is a better outcome of healing in the case of the short-term use of a splint [30].

The current trends in dentoalveolar traumatology recommend the use of a splint in cases of luxation and avulsion of a tooth and in fractures of the root and alveolar ridge [31]. **Table 1** shows basic guidelines for the use of splints, in relation to the type of trauma, the duration of mobilization, and the type of splint.

Type of trauma	Duration of immobilization	Type of splint
Subluxation	2 weeks	Flexible
Extrusive luxation	2 weeks	Flexible
Avulsion	2 weeks	Flexible
Lateral luxation	4 weeks	Flexible
Fracture of the central third of the root	4 weeks	Rigid
Fracture of the cervical third of the root	4 weeks	Rigid
Fracture of the alveolar process	4 months	Rigid

Table 1.
Recommendations for the type and duration of immobilization depending on the type of trauma.

5. Conclusions

There is a large selection of splints which are indicated for tooth trauma (**Table 2**).

Modern trends in dentoalveolar traumatology support the use of functional and flexible splints for luxation and avulsion.

	Type of splints		Indications	Contraindications	Advantages	Disadvantages
RIGID SPLINTS	**Wire ligature splints**		Mixed dentition	Generally avoided in case of availability of other methods	Useful for oral surgeons when other splinting methods are not available	Gingival irritation and inflammation
RIGID SPLINTS	**Surgical suture**		No neighboring teeth to which splint may be fixed	When other splinting methods would be better choice	Useful for oral surgeons as an alternative splint	Early suture loosening
RIGID SPLINTS	**Arch bar splint**		Jaw fractures	Dento-alveolar trauma where repair of PDL is expected	none	Gingival irritation and inflammation
RIGID SPLINTS	**Acrylic splints**		Luxation of tooth in combination with fracture of alveolar bone	Isolated dental trauma	Individual splint that can be made with direct and indirect technique	Direct method creates warm reaction
RIGID SPLINTS	**Composite splint**		When neighboring teeth are intact	Artificial crowns/ large fillings	Every dental office have it, Easy to apply	Tendency to split due to occlusal forces
SEMIRIGID/FLEXIBLE SPLINTS	**Orthodontic brackets and arches**		When injured tooth is intruded and must be repositioned later by orthodontic forces	When there is a doubt that orthodontic forces will disturb the healing process of injured tooth	Possibility of synchronizing movement of teeth	Tricky to use for non orthodontic specialist, possible irritation of the lips which can be avoid by applying the wax,
SEMIRIGID/FLEXIBLE SPLINTS	**Wire - composite splints**		All cases of traumatic injuries except for alveolar fracture	Artificial crowns/ large fillings	Easy to apply, most commonly available dento-alveolar splint	Problems with removing the splint
SEMIRIGID/FLEXIBLE SPLINTS	**Fibre splints**	Fishing line		Alveolar fracture	Easy to manipulate/apply Favorable healing outcomes	none
SEMIRIGID/FLEXIBLE SPLINTS	**Fibre splints**	Glass-ionomer fibre				
SEMIRIGID/FLEXIBLE SPLINTS	**Fibre splints**	Ribbond splints				More expensive in comparison with a wire composite splints
SEMIRIGID/FLEXIBLE SPLINTS	**Fibre splints**	Kevlar fibre				
SEMIRIGID/FLEXIBLE SPLINTS	**Titanium trauma splint**				Reduce the quantity of composite material, easy to apply and remove	High cost
Conclusion			Current trends in dento-alveolar traumatology support the use of flexible splints in all types of luxation and tooth avulsion. Rigid splints are recommended in case of a root fracture and fracture of the alveolar process. Following right indication any kind of splint is better than no splint at all			

Table 2.
Classification of splints with indications, contraindications, advantages, and disadvantages.

The prognosis for traumatized teeth is more determined by the type of trauma than the type of splint selected.

The type of splint and the duration of immobilization, therefore, may not be considered significant variables in terms of the outcome of healing.

Acknowledgements

The author would like to thank Armin Klančević, DMD, for his contribution of drawing all the figures for this chapter.

Conflict of interest

The authors declare there is no conflict of interest.

Author details

Naida Hadziabdic
Department of Oral Surgery, Faculty of Dental Medicine, University of Sarajevo, Sarajevo, Bosnia and Herzegovina

*Address all correspondence to: nsulejma@yahoo.com

References

[1] Rao A, Rao A, Shenoy R. Splinting—When and how? Dental Update. 2011;**38**:341-342, 344-6. DOI: 10.12968/denu.2011.38.5.341

[2] Andreasen JO, Ahrensburg SS, Tendal B. Inappropriate use of meta-analysis in an evidence-based assessment of the clinical guidelines for replanted avulsed teeth. Timing of pulp extirpation, splinting periods and prescription of systemic antibiotics. Dental Traumatology. 2010;**26**:451-452. DOI: 10.1111/j.1600-9657.2010.00911.x

[3] Andreasen JO, Lauridsen E, Andreasen FM. Contradictions in the treatment of traumatic dental injuries and ways to proceed in dental trauma research. Dental Traumatology. 2010;**26**:16-22. DOI: 10.1111/j.1600-9657.2009.00818.x

[4] Brown CL, Macie IC. Splinting of traumatized teeth in children. Dental Update. 2003;**30**:78-82. DOI: 10.12968/denu.2003.30.2.78

[5] Ben Hassan MW, Andersson L, Lucas PW. Stiffness characteristics of splints for fixation of traumatized teeth. Dental Traumatology. 2016;**32**:140-145. DOI: 10.1111/edt.12234

[6] Kahler B, Hu JY, Marriot-Smith CS, Heithersay GS. Splinting of teeth following trauma: A review and a new splinting recommendation. Australian Dental Journal. 2016;**61**:59-73. DOI: 10.1111/adj.12398

[7] Kahler B, Heithersay GS. An evidence-based appraisal of splinting luxated, avulsed and root-fractured teeth. Dental Traumatology. 2008;**24**:2-10. DOI: 10.1111/j.1600-9657.2006.00480.x

[8] Cho WC, Nam OH, Kim MS, Lee HS, Choi SC. A retrospective study of traumatic dental injuries in primary dentition: Treatment outcomes of splinting. Acta Odontologica Scandinavica. 2018;**76**:253-256. DOI: 10.1080/00016357.2017.1414956

[9] Malmgren B, Andreasen JO, Flores MT, Robertson A, Diangelis AJ, Andersson L, et al. International Association of Dental Traumatology guidelines for the management of traumatic dental injuries: 3. Injuries in the primary dentition. Dental Traumatology. 2012;**28**:174-182. DOI: 10.1111/j.1600-9657.2012.01146.x

[10] Andersson L, Andreasen JO, Day P, Heithersay G, Trope M, DiAngelis AJ, et al. International Association of Dental Traumatology guidelines for the management of traumatic dental injuries: 2. Avulsion of permanent teeth. Dental Traumatology. 2012;**28**:88-96. DOI: 10.1111/j.1600-9657.2012.01125.x

[11] Mazzoleni S, Meschia G, Cortesi R, Bressan E, Tomasi C, Ferro R, et al. In vitro comparison of the flexibility of different splint systems used in dental traumatology. Dental Traumatology. 2010;**26**:30-36. DOI: 10.1111/j.1600-9657.2009.00843.x

[12] Burcak Cengiz S, Stephan Atac A, Cehreli ZC. Biomechanical effects of splint types on traumatized tooth: A photoelastic stress analysis. Dental Traumatology. 2006;**22**:133-138. DOI: 10.1111/j.1600-9657.2006.00339.x

[13] Gupta S, Sharma A, Dang N. Suture splint: An alternative for luxation injuries of teeth in pediatric patients—A case report. The Journal of Clinical Pediatric Dentistry. 1997;**22**:19-21

[14] Neaverth EJ, Georig AC. Technique and rationale for splinting. Journal of the American Dental Association. 1980;**100**:56-63. DOI: 10.14219/jada.archive.1980.0026

[15] Lin S, Emodi O, Abu El-Naaj I. Splinting of an injured tooth as part

of emergency treatment. Dental Traumatology. 2008;**24**:370-372. DOI: 10.1111/j.1600-9657.2007.00530.x

[16] Lello JL, Lello GE. The effect of interdental continuous loop wire splinting and intermaxillary fixation on the marginal gingiva. International Journal of Oral and Maxillofacial Surgery. 1988;**17**:249-252. DOI: 10.1016/s0901-5027(88)80050-x

[17] Berthold C, Thaler A, Petschelt A. Rigidity of commonly used dental trauma splints. Dental Traumatology. 2009;**25**:248-255. DOI: 10.1111/j.1600-9657.2008.00683.x

[18] Oikarinen K. Comparison of the flexibility of various splinting methods for tooth fixation. International Journal of Oral and Maxillofacial Surgery. 1988;**17**:125-127. DOI: 10.1016/s0901-5027(88)80166-8

[19] Oikarinen K. Tooth splinting: A review of the literature and consideration of the versatility of a wire-composite splint. Endodontics & Dental Traumatology. 1990;**6**:237-250. DOI: 10.1111/j.1600-9657.1990.tb00426.x

[20] Alexander PC. Replantation of teeth. Oral Surgery, Oral Medicine, and Oral Pathology. 1956;**9**:110-114. DOI: 10.1016/0030-4220(56)90181-5

[21] Dawoodbhoy I, Valiathan A, Lalani ZS, Cariappa KM. Splinting of avulsed central incisors with orthodontic wires: A case report. Endodontics & Dental Traumatology. 1994;**10**:149-152. DOI: 10.1111/j.1600-9657.1994.tb00541.x

[22] Croll TP, Helpin ML. Use of self-etching adhesive system and compomer for splinting traumatized incisors. Pediatric Dentistry. n.d.;**24**:53-56

[23] von Arx T. Splinting of traumatized teeth with focus on adhesive techniques. Journal of the California Dental Association. 2005;**33**:409-414

[24] Kargul B, Caglar E, Kabalay U. Glass fiber-reinforced composite resin as fixed space maintainers in children: 12-Month clinical follow-up. Journal of Dentistry for Children (Chicago, Ill.). 2005;**72**:109-112

[25] Marriot-Smith C, Marino V, Heithersay GS. A preclinical dental trauma teaching module. Dental Traumatology. 2016;**32**:247-250. DOI: 10.1111/edt.12251

[26] Yildirim Öz G, Ataoğlu H, Kir N, Karaman AI. An alternative method for splinting of traumatized teeth: Case reports. Dental Traumatology. 2006;**22**:345-349. DOI: 10.1111/j.1600-9657.2005.00364.x

[27] Filippi A, Von Arx T, Lussi A. Comfort and discomfort of dental trauma splints—A comparison of a new device (TTS) with three commonly used splinting techniques. Dental Traumatology. 2002;**18**:275-280. DOI: 10.1034/j.1600-9657.2002.00121.x

[28] Stellini E, Avesani S, Mazzoleni S, Favero L. Laboratory comparison of a titanium trauma splint with three conventional ones for the treatment of dental trauma. European Journal of Paediatric Dentistry. 2005;**6**:191-196

[29] Von Arx T, Filippi A, Lussi A. Comparison of a new dental trauma splint device (TTS) with three commonly used splinting techniques. Dental Traumatology. 2001;**17**:266-274. DOI: 10.1034/j.1600-9657.2001.170605.x

[30] Hinckfuss SE, Messer LB. Splinting duration and periodontal outcomes for replanted avulsed teeth: A systematic review. Dental Traumatology. 2009;**25**:150-157. DOI: 10.1111/j.1600-9657.2008.00761.x

[31] Qin M, Ge L, Bai R. Use of a removable splint in the treatment of subluxated, luxated and root fractured anterior permanent teeth in children. Dental Traumatology. 2002;**18**:81-85. DOI: 10.1034/j.1600-9657.2002.180207.x

Section 2

TMJ and Maxillomandibular Lesions

Chapter 5

Medication-Related Osteonecrosis of the Jaw: An Overview

Marko Blašković and Dorotea Blašković

Abstract

Medication-related osteonecrosis of the jaw (MRONJ) is a rare side effect of medications belonging to the antiresorptive (AR) and antiangiogenic (AA) groups. The first cases were described in the literature in 2003, and more than 1300 publications and 15,000 cases have been published since then. The incidence of MRONJ among cancer patients treated with bisphosphonates is 0–6.7%, with denosumab is 0.7–1.7% and with bevacizumab is 0.2%. Patients treated for osteoporosis have a lower risk of developing MRONJ at 0.02 and 0.04% with bisphosphonates and 0.2% with denosumab. In more than 50% of cases, tooth extraction was considered the causative factor responsible for the onset of the MRONJ. Treatment strategies include preventive, medical and surgical interventions.

Keywords: medication-related osteonecrosis of the jaw, bisphosphonate-related osteonecrosis of the jaw, antiresorptive-associated osteonecrosis of the jaw, denosumab, antiangiogenic medicamentations

1. Introduction

Medication-related osteonecrosis of the jaw (MRONJ) is a side effect of some medications belonging to the antiresorptive (AR), such as bisphosphonates and denosumab, and antiangiogenic (AA) groups. The disease is present as an exposed necrotic bone in the maxilla or mandible persisting for more than 8 weeks in patients taking the aforementioned medical therapy but without a past history of radiotherapy [1, 2]. The first cases described in 2003 were thought to be a side effect of bisphosphonates (BP) alone and was termed bisphosphonate-related osteonecrosis of the jaws [3, 4]. More than 1300 publications with more than 15,000 cases have been published since then, with two new names indicating that medications other than BPs could help trigger osteonecrosis of the jaws [5].

Reports of denosumab-associated osteonecrosis began surfacing in 2010, which led the American Dental Association to revise the term 'MRONJ' to antiresorptive-related osteonecrosis of the jaws (ARONJ) to stress the fact that other antiresorptive compounds could lead to osteonecrosis of the jaws [6–11].

Recently published literature has, however, demonstrated the implication of both antiresorptive and antiangiogenic medications in osteonecrosis of the jaws. It was known previously that the antiangiogenic medications could increase the incidence of osteonecrosis of the jaws when they were administered together with BP [12, 13]. New evidence indicates that antiangiogenic therapy can cause osteonecrosis of the jaws in patients naive to BP therapy [12]. Consequently, the American Association of Oral and Maxillofacial Surgeons (AAOMS) published an update in

2014 establishing the new moniker 'MRONJ' to better reflect the variety of medications known to induce jaw osteonecrosis [14].

From a historical stand point, the first cases of the jaw osteonecrosis were described in the nineteenth century in matchmaking industry workers who were exposed to phosphorous compounds. The condition was known as 'phossy jaw', a painful jaw bone exposure associated with sequestration and infection. It was a very progressive condition with high mortality rate because of the absence of antibiotic therapy. The incidence of the condition "phossy jaw" decreased significantly due to the improvement of the working conditions in the matchmaking industry [15].

In the literature, this condition is known under several names and acronyms:

MRONJ—medication-related osteonecrosis of the jaw
BRONJ—bisphosphonate-related osteonecrosis of the jaw
BAONJ—bisphosphonate-associated osteonecrosis of the jaw
ARONJ—antiresorptive-associated osteonecrosis of the jaw
BON—bisphosphonate osteonecrosis
ONJ—osteonecrosis of the jaw [5]

1.1 Antiresorptive medicaments: bisphosphonates (BPs)

Bisphosphonates belong to a group of antiresorptive medications often used to treat osteoporosis. Other members of the AR group are monoclonal antibodies against receptor activator of nuclear factor-κ denosumab (RANKL), selective oestrogen receptor modulators, estrogens and calcitonin. Only the first two members, BP and denosumab, are associated with MRONJ. Unfortunately, these are also the most commonly utilised medications for the treatment of osteoporosis. BPs are in fact considered the first-choice treatment for osteoporosis worldwide [16, 17].

The first biological use of BP dates back to the 1960s, when etidronate was used to treat heterotopic ossification. Soon after, further research led to the use of BP in the treatment of osteoporosis [18, 19]. BPs are also used to treat non-malignant diseases affecting the bone tissue such as Paget's disease of bone, fibrous dysplasia, cystic fibrosis, primary hyperparathyroidism and osteogenesis imperfecta [19–23].

They are also used to treat osseous malignant conditions such as metastases of solid tumours, malignant hypercalcemia and multiple myeloma. The literature shows that BPs have significant positive effects on the quality of life in cancer patients by reducing complications such as bone fractures, pain and serum calcium imbalances. Furthermore, some members of the BP family such as zolendronate also present antiangiogenic and antitumour features by inhibiting human endothelial cell proliferation and changes in endothelial cell migration and adhesion. Zolendronate's antitumour effects include induction of apoptosis as well as inhibition of cell invasion and adhesion. These aforementioned features are beneficial in delaying tumour growth [17, 24–29].

BPs can be divided into two groups based on the presence or absence of nitrogen atom in the side chain. The presence of nitrogen is related to the higher potency of the BP, which will clinically translate to a better antiresorptive effect and higher binding affinity to hydroxyapatite within bones. It is estimated that BPs have half lives in bone of approximately 11 years [30, 31]. Unfortunately, higher potency of the medication is also linked to a higher incidence of MRONJ. Bone resorption is achieved by two mechanisms. Non-nitrogen BPs are linked to osteoclast apoptosis. Nitrogen-containing BPs have a much more complex working mechanism that inhibits mevalonate signalling to impact osteoclastogenesis, apoptosis and cytoskeletal dynamics [32].

1.2 Antiresorptive medicaments: denosumab

Denosumab is a human monoclonal antibody that inhibits receptor-activated nuclear factor-κB ligand (RANKL). Denosumab prevents the RANKL activation, which is crucial for osteoclast activation, function and differentiation resulting in decreased bone resorption and cancer-induced bone destruction [33–37]. It is available under two names: Prolia, which is used for treating osteoporosis, and Xgeva, which is used for treating complications in patients with bone metastases and solid tumours. The dosing used in the treatment of osteoporosis is 60 mg subcutaneous injection every 6 months. The treatment of patients with bone metastasis is 120 mg subcutaneous injection every 4 weeks [37]. Although the incidence of MRONJ is similar in patients treated with BPs and denosumab, there are some advantages of denosumab over bisphosphonates such as improved efficacy and better tolerability. Furthermore, denosumab creates no nephrotoxic effects and may be used in patients with renal insufficiency [36, 38, 39].

2. Antiangiogenic medications

Antiangiogenic medicines are used to treat patients with different types of tumours such as gastrointestinal stromal tumour, glioblastoma, hepatocellular carcinoma, hormone receptor-positive breast carcinoma, mantle cell lymphoma, metastatic colorectal carcinoma, multiple myeloma, metastatic renal cell carcinoma, non-squamous non-small cell lung carcinoma, pancreatic neuroendocrine tumour, renal cell carcinoma, subependymal giant cell astrocytoma and soft tissue sarcoma. They are used to inhibit or decrease neoangiogenesis which is crucial for the expansive tumour growth. It was known previously that antiangiogenic medications could increase the incidence of osteonecrosis of the jaws when administered concurrently with BP or denosumab [12, 40–43]. New evidence indicates that antiangiogenic therapy can also cause osteonecrosis of the jaws in patients naive to BP therapy [12, 41, 42, 44–49]. Many AA-associated cases of MRONJ were reported after the use of sunitinib and sorafenib, both of which are members of tyrosine kinase inhibitors [37].

3. Diagnosis of the MRONJ

In order to diagnose MRONJ, three diagnostic factors must be met:

1. Current or previous treatment with antiresorptive and/or antiangiogenic agents

2. Exposed bone or bone that can be probed through an intraoral or extraoral fistula in the maxillofacial region that has persisted for more than 8 weeks

3. No history of radiation therapy to the jaws or obvious metastatic disease to the jaws [1, 7, 14, 50]

Radiation therapy of the jaws must be excluded since the clinical presentation of the osteoradionecrosis and MRONJ may be impossible to distinguish. A diagnosis of osteoradionecrosis should be considered in patients with the aforementioned symptoms as well as a history of head or neck radiotherapy [7].

MRONJ diagnosis is established mainly via oral examination and review of medical history. Other more complex diagnostic tools such as imaging modalities or histopathological examinations are not specific enough and should be used as adjunctive tools to assess the stage and extent of the disease. The initial diagnosis of MRONJ can be made by any dentist or physician with a basic understanding of MRONJ [7, 50].

Consultations with the patient's physician are critical because many patients remain confused or forgetful regarding their current or previous antiresorptive/antiangiogenic therapy. Furthermore, cancer patients may receive a complex therapy consisting of different medications used at different time sequences, which contributes to the overall confusion.

3.1 Clinical picture of MRONJ

A defining feature of MRONJ is the exposure of necrotic bone or fistulation that can be probed to the osseous surface which fails to heal for more than 8 weeks. This clinical finding can be anticipated by mild pain and discomfort in the affected site. As the disease progresses, the adjacent soft tissue becomes inflamed, appearing erythematosus and swollen. Purulent exudate may be present as a consequence of a secondary infection. In the later stages of the disease, oroantral fistula, oronasal fistula, oral cutaneous fistula or pathological fractures may be present [1, 7, 14, 51].

3.2 Imaging

Radiographic features of MRONJ are not pathognomonic and depend on the stage and development of the disease.

In the early stages of the disease, zones of higher and diffused radiopacity and thickening of the lamina dura can be present within the affected bone. Previous extraction sites may demonstrate minimal or complete absence of bone healing, which results in radiolucent radiographic appearance with a prominent residual lamina dura.

In more developed stages of MRONJ, the exposed bone becomes colonised by bacteria which induce focal bone demineralisation. Radiography shows a poorly circumscribed mixture of radiolucent and radiopaque zones. Other osteolytic processes with similar radiographic findings include osteomyelitis, multiple myeloma, metastatic disease and primary lymphoma of the bone [7, 52].

Further advancement of the disease can result in the formation of bony sequestra, which is visible on radiographic image as radiopaque or mottled fragments surrounded by a radiolucent border. Additionally, in some cancer patients treated with BP, a periosteal thickening (mimicking a second layer of compact bone surrounding the cortical bone) and new bone formation on the Schneiderian mucous membrane were described [7, 52, 53].

MRI and Technetium-99m imaging modalities may be more useful in detecting the presence of inflammation in patients with established MRONJ [7].

Scintigraphy may show additional benefits in cancer patients undergoing intravenous (IV) BP therapy. There exists evidence that many of those who presented with an increased tracer uptake in the jaws subsequently developed necrosis, though further research is needed to confirm these findings [54, 55].

PET imaging has low diagnostic values in MRONJ because of a low level of sensitivity and accuracy [7].

3.3 Histopathology

MRONJ specimens are composed of grey coloured hard tissue and, occasionally, friable soft tissue. Decalcification of the larger specimens can be prolonged as a result of bone sclerosis. In contrast, smaller bone specimens may have soft consistency as a result of bacterial colonisation. While the necrotic fragments are devoid of osteocytes and osteoclasts, they may have bacterial debris adherent to their surfaces from bone exposure. The adjacent soft tissue consists of granulation tissue with or without abscess formation [7, 52].

Although infrequently, metastatic cancer was identified in bone specimens clinically diagnosed as MRONJ in cancer patients exposed to BP therapy. Thus, all the bone specimens obtained from MRONJ cancer patients either by biopsy, sequestrectomy or segmental osteotomy should be sent for histopathological analysis [56].

3.4 Microbiology

Microbiological culture assessment of exposed bone has previously failed to identify a definite, specific microbial aetiology behind MRONJ. The samples demonstrated a polymicrobial infection caused by pathogens present in the normal oral flora [7, 52].

4. Frequency of MRONJ

MRONJ is an uncommon disease whose frequency is generally low regardless of the type of antiresorptive or antiangiogenic medications administered. According to one study, an average general dentist can expect one new case of MRONJ every 62 years of his work among patients on oral BP [57]. The overall risk of MRONJ among patients with cancer diagnosis (primary or metastatic) is 0–6.7% if treated with IV BPs [58–60], 0.7–1.7% if treated with denosumab [58, 61, 62] and 0.2% if treated with the AA agent bevacizumab [12, 58, 63]. The risk range of MRONJ among patients who are exposed to both zolendronate (intravenous BP) and bevacizumab (antiangiogenic) is 0.9% [12]. The risk among patients treated for osteoporosis who are exposed to oral zolendronate alone is 0.02% [58, 64], while the risk for patients treated with denosumab alone is 0.04–0.2% [58, 65, 66].

5. Risk factors of MRONJ

5.1 Risk factors connected with AR medications

- Route of administration of AR medications

  Patients with intraosseous malignancies are treated intravenously with BP or subcutaneously with denosumab, while patients affected with osteoporosis can be treated with oral or intravenous BP medications or subcutaneously with denosumab.

  Oral BPs are associated with lower occurrence risk of MRONJ than intravenous BPs or denosumab. The incidence of AR therapy-associated MRONJ is significantly lower for osteoporosis patients than for cancer patients [58].

- Duration of BP therapy

  The prevalence of MRONJ increases over time, from 0.5 to 0.6% after 1 year of therapy, 0.9 to 1.1% after 2 years and 1.3 to 1.1% after 3 years [67]. For patients with osteoporosis who are exposed to oral BPs, the prevalence of MRONJ increases over time from 0 to 0.2% after 4 years. The average duration of BP therapy in patients who developed MRONJ is 4.4 years [58]. Some authors found that there were no significant increases in risk between the third and fourth years of BP therapy [59].

- Dose and potency

Zoledronic acid is considered the most potent BP medication. Its potency is estimated to be 10 times higher compared to ibandronate and 20 times higher than pamidronate [68].

5.2 Local factors

- Dental treatment

Dentoalveolar surgery with bone manipulation (tooth extraction, implant placement and periodontal or endodontic surgical procedures) is the most common local risk factor for patients exposed to AR/AA with MRONJ. Tooth extraction was considered a precipitating factor in 52–61% of cases of MRONJ. In addition, exposure to zolendronate prior to tooth extraction incurred a 16- to 33-fold increase in risk of MRONJ [13, 69, 70]. The risk for patients treated with oral BPs is 0.5% or less [71, 72]. The same risk for the cancer patients treated with intravenous BPs is within the range of 1.6–14.8% [73, 74] or 1.7–4.7% [72] depending on the investigation.

Though they are considered risk factors, the exact rate of MRONJ in patients treated with AA/AR medications after periodontal, implant or endodontic surgeries is not yet certain. Anecdotal experience stipulates that they nonetheless demonstrate similar risks when compared to dental extractions [14].

- Dental or implant inflammation

The inflammatory processes associated with dentoalveolar surgery are considered a causative factor in developing MRONJ. The periodontal or periapical pathology were considered a risk factor for 50% of the cases of MRONJ [13, 14, 73, 75, 76]. Since many dental inflammatory diseases are treated via extraction, the exact degree to which surgical trauma or inflammatory changes actually contribute to the development of osteonecrosis is not yet clear [27].

5.3 Anatomic factors

MRONJ appears in the mandible more often than in the maxilla. Instance in the lower jaw is 73%, in upper jaw is 22.5% and in both jaws is 4.5% [13, 14].

Denture use increases the risk of MRONJ. This is especially true in cases of cancer patients with dentures exposed to ibandronate, zolendronate or pamidronate. These patients experience a two-fold increase in risk of osteonecrosis [69, 70].

5.4 Demographic risk factors

Higher prevalence of MRONJ in the female population may be associated with the prevalence of osteolytic conditions in women [14]. Women over 50 have a 50 and 12% lifetime risk of developing osteoporosis and breast cancer, respectively.

On the other hand, men in the same age group have a 20% risk of developing osteoporosis and a 17% risk of prostate cancer [16].

Few studies have been conducted exploring MRONJ risk in the paediatric population. However, a recent survey of the literature revealed no significant rate of MRONJ despite the fact that a number of patients were exposed to long-lasting BP therapies and invasive dental treatments [77, 78].

5.5 Systemic risk factors

Corticosteroids [13, 75] and antiangiogenic [12, 13, 37, 40–43, 45–49, 69] medications may increase the risk of MRONJ when administered concurrently with a bisphosphonate.

Other comorbidities were inconsistently linked to elevated risk of developing MRONJ, such as anaemia, diabetes [13, 75] and the type of cancer [15, 16].

6. Staging of MRONJ

The staging system was developed primarily to guide the clinician with specific treatment strategies according to clinical presentation. Furthermore, it helped introduce homogeneity to MRONJ literature, allowing for new advancements in the diagnosis and treatment of the disease.

The guidelines were first published in 2006 then updated in 2009 and 2014 as a result of new findings relevant for treatment of the disease [2, 7, 14].

6.1 Stage 0

The initial stage includes patients exposed to AR/AA therapy with no clinical evidence of exposed or necrotic bone. Only non-specific symptoms are present which cannot be attributed to other pathological entities. Recent literature suggests that up to 50% of patients at stage 0 will progress to the subsequent stage.

1. **Symptoms present during stage 0**: odontalgia not explained by dental cause, dull pain in the body of the mandible, sinus pain and altered neurosensory function.

2. **Clinical findings present during stage 0**: increased tooth mobility not explained by periodontal disease and fistula that is not associated with endodontic pathology.

3. **Radiographic findings present during stage 0**: alveolar bone resorption not associated with periodontal disease, thickening of the maxillary sinus walls, irregular trabecular patterns, absence of bone healing and persistent lamina dura in extraction sites, thickening of the lamina dura and a decrease in the size of the periodontal ligament space.

6.2 Stage 1

The clinical picture of stage 1 consists of exposed necrotic bone or a fistula that can be probed to the bone. Since there is no infection, the patients typically do not experience additional symptoms. Radiographic findings mentioned in the stage 0 may also be present.

6.3 Stage 2

In the second stage, the exposed necrotic bone is infected and the patients experience pain. Second stage patients can present with abscess and fistulation as well. Radiographic findings mentioned in the stage 0 may also be present. The adjacent soft tissues may be swollen or secondarily infected.

6.4 Stage 3

All of the symptoms and clinical findings characteristic of the second stage are also present in the third stage: infection, pain and exposed necrotic bone or fistulation that probes to bone. Furthermore, one or more of the following symptoms manifest as a result of disease progression beyond the anatomical borders of the alveolar bone:

- Exposed necrotic bone reaching the inferior border of the mandible or the floor of the maxillary sinuses
- Pathological fracture
- Extra-oral fistula
- Oroantral or oronasal communication
- Bone resorption extending to the inferior border of the mandible or the sinus floor [7, 14, 52]

7. Treatment of MRONJ

Three different types of treatment strategies have been developed for the MRONJ: preventive, [79, 80] medical and surgical treatments [14, 81]. Preventive measures are indicated for patients who are slated for AA/AR therapy or have undergone treatment without notable symptoms of MRONJ. The latter two treatment modalities are used to treat patients with an established diagnosis of MRONJ.

7.1 Preventing MRONJ

Preventive measures are undertaken to reduce risk factors and preserve oral health of the patient at risk of developing MRONJ. The incidence of MRONJ can be reduced by up to one third if preventive measures are applied. These measures differ depending on the indications of the AR/AA therapy as well as the nature of the triggering dental treatment.

Preventive measures fundamentally rely on proper communication and collaboration between the oncologist, the primary care physician, the dentist and the patient. The healthcare professionals must inform the patient of the possibility of developing MRONJ and of the importance of oral health in its prevention. Prior to initiating AR/AA treatment, the patient should be referred to a dentist for a complete clinical and radiological oral examination. It is the dentist's responsibility to evaluate the risk factors (such as dental decay, periodontal diseases and ill-fitting prostheses) for each individual patient, eliminate or decrease the risk factors, restore oral health and maintain oral health throughout and after the AA/AR treatment [79, 80].

According to some studies, only 30% of the patients taking BP are referred to a dentist because of a lack of AR/AA prescriber awareness. In addition, approximately 40–50% of dentists expressed a low-to-moderate level of knowledge of MRONJ, sometimes requesting discontinuation of medications not associated with osteonecrosis of the jaw [82, 83].

7.1.1 Cancer patients with AR/AA therapy

Before initiating AA/AR treatment, the oncologist should inform the patient about possible oral side effects and refer the patient to a dentist for comprehensive dental examination [79, 80]. Dentoalveolar surgery remains the major risk factor for developing MRONJ and extraction increases this risk, as do periodontal or periapical pathology [13, 69, 70]. As estimated above, pre-existing dental inflammatory disease is a risk factor for more than 50% of cases [13, 14, 73, 75, 76]. Thus, in accordance with the oncologists, the onset of the AR/AA therapy should be postponed until dental health is established. All extractions and dentoalveolar surgery should be performed and the surgical sites should be allowed to heal completely. Some studies advise at least 2–3 weeks of mucosal healing, while others recommend up to 45–60 days prior to initiation of AA/AR therapy [14, 79]. In the case of patients with total or partial dentures, intraoral examination for decubital areas should be performed. Old or ill-fitting dentures should be relined or replaced [69, 70].

If a cancer patient has already been exposed to AR/AA compounds, preventive therapy is directed towards preventing infections and avoiding dentoalveolar surgery. Consequently, good oral hygiene and frequent recalls are of paramount importance. All infected dentition should be addressed via endodontic therapy. If surgery cannot be avoided, chlorhexidine (CHX) mouth wash 0.12% should be started 7 days before the surgical procedure 2–3 times per day and should be continued for the next 2 weeks after the extraction. Antibiotic treatment should also be initiated before the extraction and continued afterwards, though there exists no current consensus [79] on the type, duration, onset and route of administration of the antibiotic therapy [84]. Some authors also recommend deep scaling of the remaining teeth prior to surgical interventions [72].

Again, proper communication must be established between the oncologist, the dentist and the patient to reduce the rate of complications.

7.1.2 Osteoporosis patients with AR/AA therapy

The risk of MRONJ in osteoporosis patients on oral bisphosphonate therapy increases significantly when the duration of therapy exceeds 4 years. During the first 4 years of oral BP therapy, minor surgical procedures can typically be performed without therapy modification. Thus, prophylactic dentoalveolar surgery is not critical to the degree it is in cancer patients and/or those undergoing IV AR/AA therapies. The patient should nonetheless be monitored regularly and given proper oral hygiene instruction [14, 79].

Patients who have been prescribed with a combination of BP, AA or corticosteroids demonstrate an additive risk of developing MRONJ [12, 13, 37, 40–43, 45–49, 69]. There exists much discussion in the literature regarding discontinuation (drug holiday) of BP therapy prior to surgical procedures. The purpose of a 'drug holiday' is to reduce the risk of MRONJ and complications with wound healing. However, suspension of BPs may increase the risk of complications including fractures. Furthermore, BPs have long half-lives when bound to hydroxyapatite, and the efficacy of a temporary discontinuation has been questioned. The clinician must weigh the risk of MRONJ with the risk of complications in partnership with the physician who prescribed the BP therapy [1, 11, 14, 79, 84].

According to the guidelines from the AAOMS, a pre-operative drug holiday of 2 months may be considered regardless of the total duration of BP therapy. This should also be done in partnership with the physician who has prescribed the BP therapy. All BP therapy should be resumed once all appropriate post-operative healing has occurred [14].

7.2 Medical management of MRONJ

The aim of medical management is to prevent infection of the exposed bone using topical or systemic antibiotics. The use of analgesics is indicated if the patient complains of odontalgia or dull pain located in the affected areas. Since more than 50% of patients diagnosed with stage 0 progress to a higher stage, frequent recalls with oral health instructions and preventive measure can be beneficial in the long term [54, 81, 85].

Patients presenting with stage 0 and 1 of MRONJ may be treated with medical modalities only. Adjunctive therapy is used to enhance healing of the exposed bone by decreasing inflammation, improving vascularization and stimulating bone turnover.

- Typically, the topical antibiotic of choice is chlorhexidine gluconate 0.12%

- Systemic antibiotics

  The first line antibiotic is a penicillin-class antibiotic such as amoxicillin. In case of allergy, clindamycin, fluoroquinolones and/or metronidazole may be used. Currently, there exists no scientific consensus on the duration of antibiotic therapy, though an empiric proposition recommends a 2-week course for patients with a persistent stage 1 disease and 4–6 weeks course therapy for more advanced stages of the disease.

- Pentoxifylline and vitamin E

  The combinations of these drugs have already found some success in the treatment of osteoradionecrosis. Their specific mechanism of action in the treatment of MRONJ is not completely understood. It is believed that their ability to decrease inflammation and promote vascularization can contribute to positive outcomes. Though the duration of the treatment has not been established, some studies recommend suspension of this therapy after 3 years. Patients with all stages of osteonecrosis may benefit from pentoxifylline and vitamin E. The recommended dose of pentoxifylline is 400 mg twice daily and 1000 IU vitamin E daily.

- Teriparatide

  This drug is used primarily in the treatment of osteoporosis. It may improve bone remodelling by stimulating osteoblasts, increasing bone cell signalling and activating osteoclasts. The safety, side effects, dosing and duration of the therapy for MRONJ are currently not known and additional research is warranted.

- Hyperbaric oxygen therapy

  Hyperbaric oxygen therapy is used in the treatment of osteoradionecrosis because of its purported beneficial effects on wound healing. This treatment may help provide greater oxygenation to tissues with reduced vascular supplies, accelerating wound healing and increasing bone turnover. Currently, the clinical utility of hyperbaric oxygen therapy in the treatment of MRONJ remains unclear. Higher costs and extended therapy duration could prevent routine use in MRONJ therapy [81].

7.3 Surgical treatment of MRONJ

Surgical treatment is typically indicated for the second and third stages of the disease. The degree of surgical intervention can vary from simple sequestrectomy to marginal or segmental osteotomies depending on disease dissemination, patient comorbidities, medical status and treatment expectations.

Mobile bone sequestra should always be removed regardless of the disease stage.

The term 'marginal resection' refers to surgical removal of the necrotic alveolar bone, preserving the inferior border of the mandible. On the other hand, segmental resection osteotomy includes removal of the inferior border of the mandible and results in a continuity defect. The former intervention may be used in the treatment of second stage MRONJ since the disease is limited to the alveolar bone. Consequently, the latter is reserved for the third stage of the disease as it is characterised by progression beyond the anatomical borders of the alveolar bone.

During surgical extractions or alveoplasties, the soft tissue over the bone defect should be sutured in multiple layers to ensure primary intention healing. Pre- and post-op systemic antibiotics should also be considered especially if the patient already has an established diagnosis of MRONJ [81].

Other adjunctive treatment modalities include platelet-rich fibrin (PRF) or other platelet concentrates as well as low level laser therapy. Platelet concentrates may aid soft tissue healing while low level laser therapy is linked to increased vascularity and osteoblastic differentiation, resulting in better bone healing [72, 86, 87, 89, 90].

Benefits of adjunctive treatments nonetheless remain controversial. Conflicting rates of healing have been reported when additional treatments were combined with surgical treatment compared to surgical treatments alone [86, 88–90].

8. Conclusion

MRONJ is an uncommon disease that can cause significant impairments and reductions in a patient's quality of life. Additional investments should be made to raise awareness and increase collaboration among patients, AR/AA prescribers and dentists. Issues that require further investigation include the exact number of medications associated with MRONJ, the role of drug holidays in its prevention and the choice of modalities (such as antibiotics, pentoxifylline, teriparatide and surgery) in its treatment.

Author details

Marko Blašković[1,2]* and Dorotea Blašković[2]

1 Department of Oral Surgery, Medical University of Rijeka, Rijeka, Croatia

2 Private Practice, Rijeka, Croatia

*Address all correspondence to: marko_blaskovic@yahoo.com

References

[1] Khan AA, Morrison A, Hanley DA, Felsenberg D, McCauley LK, O'Ryan F, et al. Diagnosis and management of osteonecrosis of the jaw: A systematic review and international consensus. Journal of Bone and Mineral Research. 2015;**30**(1):3-23. DOI: 10.1002/jbmr.2405

[2] Ruggiero SL, Dodson TB, Assael LA, Landesberg R, Marx RE, Mehrotra B, et al. American Association of Oral and dMaxillofacial Surgeons position paper on bisphosphonate-related osteonecrosis of the jaws—2009 update. Journal of Oral and Maxillofacial Surgery. 2009;**67**:2-12. DOI: 10.1016/j.joms.2009.01.009

[3] Marx RE. Pamidronate (Aredia) and zoledronate (Zometa) induced avascular necrosis of the jaws: A growing epidemic. Journal of Oral and Maxillofacial Surgery. 2003;**61**: 1115-1117

[4] Ruggiero SL, Mehrotra B, Rosenberg TJ, Engroff SL. Osteonecrosis of the jaws associated with the use of bisphosphonates: A review of 63 cases. Journal of Oral and Maxillofacial Surgery. 2004;**62**:527-534

[5] Marx RE. A decade of bisphosphonate bone complications: What it has taught us about bone physiology. The International Journal of Oral & Maxillofacial Implants. 2014;**29**:e247-e258. DOI: 10.11607/jomi.te61

[6] Anghaloo T, Hazboun R, Tetradis S. Pathophysiology of osteonecrosis of the jaws. Oral and Maxillofacial Surgery Clinics of North America. 2015;**27**(4):489-496. DOI: 10.1016/j.coms.2015.06.001

[7] Ruggerio SL. Diagnosis and staging of medication-related osteonecrosis of the jaw. Oral and Maxillofacial Surgery Clinics of North America. 2015;**27**(4):479-487. DOI: 10.1016/j.coms.2015.06.008

[8] Taylor K, Middlefell L, Mizen K. Osteonecrosis of the jaws induced by anti-RANK ligand therapy. The British Journal of Oral & Maxillofacial Surgery. 2010;**48**(3):221-223. DOI: 10.1016/j.bjoms.2009.08.030

[9] Anghallo T, Fenselfeld A, Tetradis S. Osteonecrosis of the jaw in patients on denosumab. Journal of Oral and Maxillofacial Surgery. 2010;**68**:959-963. DOI: 10.1016/j.joms.2009.10.010

[10] Kygridis A, Toulis KA. Denosumab-related osteonecrosis of the jaws. Osteoporosis International. 2011;**22**(1):369-370. DOI: 10.1007/s00198-010-1177-6

[11] Hellstein JW, Adler RA, Edwards B, Jacobsen PL, Kalmar JR, Koka S, et al. Managing the care of patients receiving antiresorptive therapy for prevention and treatment of osteoporosis: Executive summary of recommendations from the American Dental Association Council on Scientific Affairs. Journal of the American Dental Association (1939). 2011;**142**:1243-1251

[12] Guarneri V, Miles D, Robert N, Diéras V, Glaspy J, Smith I, et al. Bevacizumab and osteonecrosis of the jaw: Incidence and association with bisphosphonate therapy in three large prospective trials in advanced breast cancer. Breast Cancer Research and Treatment. 2010;**122**:181-188. DOI: 10.1007/s10549-010-0866-3

[13] Saad F, Brown JE, Van Poznak C, Ibrahim T, Stemmer SM, Stopeck AT, et al. Incidence, risk factors, and outcomes of osteonecrosis of the jaw: Integrated analysis from three blinded active-controlled phase III trials in cancer patients with bone metastases.

Annals of Oncology. 2012;**23**:1341-1347. DOI: 10.1093/annonc/mdr435

[14] Ruggiero SL, Dodson TB, Fantasia J, Goodday R, Aghaloo T, Mehrotra B, et al. American Association of Oral and Maxillofacial Surgeons position paper on medication-related osteonecrosis of the jaw—2014 update. Journal of Oral and Maxillofacial Surgery. 2014;**72**:1938-1956. DOI: 10.1016/j.joms.2014.04.031

[15] Hellstein JW, Marek CL. Bisphosphonate osteochemonecrosis (bis-phossy jaw): Is this phossy jaw of the 21st century? Journal of Oral and Maxillofacial Surgery. 2005;**63**:682-689. DOI: 10.1016/j.joms.2005.01.010

[16] Weinerman S, Usera GL. Antiresorptive therapies for osteoporosis. Oral and Maxillofacial Surgery Clinics of North America. 2015;**27**:555-560. DOI: 10.1016/j.coms.2015.07.001

[17] Russell RG, Xia Z, Dunford JE, Oppermann U, Kwaasi A, Hulley PA, et al. Bisphosphonates: An update on mechanisms of action and how these relate to clinical efficacy. Annals of the New York Academy of Sciences. 2007;**1117**:209-257. DOI: 10.1196/annals.1402.089

[18] Rosen CJ. A tale of two worlds in prescribing etidronate for osteoporosis. Lancet. 1997;**8**(350):1340. DOI: 10.1016/S0140-6736(05)65132-X

[19] Ruggiero SL. Bisphosphonate-related osteonecrosis of the jaw (BRONJ): Initial discovery and subsequent development. Journal of Oral and Maxillofacial Surgery. 2009;**67**(5 Suppl):13-18. DOI: 10.1016/j.joms.2008.10.005

[20] Eastell R, Walsh JS, Watts NB, Siris E. Bisphosphonates for postmenopausal osteoporosis. Bone. 2011;**49**:82-88. DOI: 10.1016/j.bone.2011.02.011

[21] Villa JC, Gianakos A, Lane JM. Bisphosphonate treatment in osteoporosis: Optimal duration of therapy and the incorporation of a drug holiday. HSS Journal. 2016;**12**:66-73. DOI: 10.1007/s11420-015-9469-1

[22] Muschitz C, Feichtinger X, Haschka J, Kocijan R. Diagnosis and treatment of Paget's disease of bone : A clinical practice guideline. Wiener Medizinische Wochenschrift (1946). 2017;**167**:18-24. DOI: 10.1007/s10354-016-0502-x

[23] Abdelmoula LC, Ben M'barek R, Ben Hadj Yahia C, Tekaya R, Testouri N, Chaabouni L, et al. Bisphosphonates: Indications in bone diseases other than osteoporosis. La Tunisie Médicale. 2011;**89**:511-516

[24] Coleman RE, McCloskey EV. Bisphosponates in oncology. Bone. 2011;**49**(1):71-76. DOI: 10.1016/j.bone.2011.02.003

[25] Mehrotra B. Antiresorptive therapies for the treatment of malignant osteolytic bone disease. Oral and Maxillofacial Surgery Clinics of North America. 2015;**27**:561-566. DOI: 10.1016/j.coms.2015.07.002

[26] Migliorati CA, Casiglia J, Epstein J, Jacobsen PL, Siegel MA, Woo SB. Managing the care of patients with bisphosphonate-associated osteonecrosis: An American Academy of Oral Medicine position paper. Journal of the American Dental Association (1939). 2005;**136**:1658-1668

[27] Body JJ, Lortholary A, Romieu G, Vigneron AM, Ford J. A dose-finding study of zoledronate in hypercalcemic cancer patients. Journal of Bone and Mineral Research. 1999;**14**:1557-1561. DOI: 10.1359/jbmr.1999.14.9.1557

[28] Hortobagyi GN, Theriault RL, Lipton A, Porter L, Blayney D, Sinoff C, et al. Long-term prevention of skeletal complications of metastatic

breast cancer with pamidronate. Protocol 19 Aredia Breast Cancer study group. Journal of Clinical Oncology. 1998;**16**:2038-2044. DOI: 10.1200/JCO.1998.16.6.2038

[29] Berenson JR, Lichtenstein A, Porter L, Dimopoulos MA, Bordoni R, George S, et al. Long-term pamidronate treatment of advanced multiple myeloma patients reduces skeletal events. Myeloma Aredia Study Group. Journal of Clinical Oncology. 1998;**16**:593-602. DOI: 10.1200/JCO.1998.16.2.593

[30] Lasseter KC, Porras AG, Denker A, Santhanagopal A, Daifotis A. Pharmacokinetic considerations in determining the terminal elimination half-lives of bisphosphonates. Clinical Drug Investigation. 2005;**25**:107-114. DOI: 10.2165/00044011-200525020-00003

[31] Fleisch H. Bisphosphonates: Mechanisms of action. Endocrine Reviews. 1998;**19**:80-100. DOI: 10.1210/edrv.19.1.0325

[32] Kimmel DB. Mechanism of action, pharmacokinetic and pharmacodynamic profile, and clinical applications of nitrogen-containing bisphosphonates. Journal of Dental Research. 2007;**86**:1022-1033. DOI: 10.1177/154405910708601102

[33] Delmas PD. Clinical potential of RANKL inhibition for the management of postmenopausal osteoporosis and other metabolic bone diseases. Journal of Clinical Densitometry. 2008;**11**:325-338. DOI: 10.1016/j.jocd.2008.02.002

[34] Cummings SR, San Martin J, McClung MR, Siris ES, Eastell R, Reid IR, et al. Denosumab for prevention of fractures in postmenopausal women with osteoporosis. The New England Journal of Medicine. 2009;**361**(8):756-765. DOI: 10.1056/NEJMoa0809493

[35] Bridgeman MB, Pathak R. Denosumab for the reduction of bone loss in postmenopausal osteoporosis: A review. Clinical Therapeutics. 2011;**33**:1547-1559. DOI: 10.1016/j.clinthera.2011.10.008

[36] Brown-Glaberman U, Stopeck AT. Role of denosumab in the management of skeletal complications in patients with bone metastases from solid tumors. Biologics. 2012;**6**:89-99. DOI: 10.2147/BTT.S20677

[37] Fantasia JE. The role of antiangiogenic therapy in the development of osteonecrosis of the jaw. Oral and Maxillofacial Surgery Clinics of North America. 2015;**27**:547-553. DOI: 10.1016/j.coms.2015.06.004

[38] Stopeck AT, Fizazi K, Body JJ, Brown JE, Carducci M, Diel I, et al. Safety of long-term denosumab therapy: Results from the open label extension phase of two phase 3 studies in patients with metastatic breast and prostate cancer. Supportive Care in Cancer. 2016;**24**:447-455. DOI: 10.1007/s00520-015-2904-5

[39] Ford JA, Jones R, Elders A, Mulatero C, Royle P, Sharma P, et al. Denosumab for treatment of bone metastases secondary to solid tumours: Systematic review and network meta-analysis. European Journal of Cancer. 2013;**49**:416-430. DOI: 10.1016/j.ejca.2012.07.016

[40] Serra E, Paolantonio M, Spoto G, Mastrangelo F, Tetè S, Dolci M. Bevacizumab-related osteneocrosis of the jaw. International Journal of Immunopathology and Pharmacology. 2009;**22**:1121-1123. DOI: 10.1177/039463200902200429

[41] Christodoulou C, Pervena A, Klouvas G, Galani E, Falagas ME, Tsakalos G, et al. Combination of bisphosphonates and antiangiogenic factors induces osteonecrosis of the jaw

more frequently than bisphosphonates alone. Oncology. 2009;**76**:209-211. DOI: 10.1159/000201931

[42] Ayllon J, Launay-Vacher V, Medioni J, Cros C, Spano JP, Oudard S. Osteonecrosis of the jaw under bisphosphonate and antiangiogenic therapies: Cumulative toxicity profile? Annals of Oncology. 2009;**20**:600-601. DOI: 10.1093/annonc/mdn788

[43] Bozas G, Roy A, Ramasamy V, Maraveyas A. Osteonecrosis of the jaw after a single bisphosphonate infusion in a patient with metastatic renal cancer treated with sunitinib. Onkologie. 2010;**33**:321-323. DOI: 10.1159/000313680

[44] Nicolatou-Galitis O, Kouri M, Papadopoulou E, Vardas E, Galiti D, Epstein JB, et al. Osteonecrosis of the jaw related to non-antiresorptive medications: A systematic review. Supportive Care in Cancer. 2018 Oct:23. DOI: 10.1007/s00520-018-4501-x

[45] Hoefert S, Eufinger H. Sunitinib may raise the risk of bisphosphonate-related osteonecrosis of the jaw: Presentation of three cases. Oral Surgery, Oral Medicine, Oral Pathology, Oral Radiology, and Endodontics. 2010;**110**:463-469. DOI: 10.1016/j.tripleo.2010.04.049

[46] Hopp RN, Pucci J, Santos-Silva AR, Jorge J. Osteonecrosis after administration of intravitreous bevacizumab. Journal of Oral and Maxillofacial Surgery. 2012;**70**:632-635. DOI: 10.1016/j.joms.2011.02.104

[47] Brunamonti Binello P, Bandelloni R, Labanca M, Buffoli B, Rezzani R, Rodella LF. Osteonecrosis of the jaws and bevacizumab therapy: A case report. International Journal of Immunopathology and Pharmacology. 2012;**25**:789-791

[48] Koch FP, Walter C, Hansen T, Jäger E, Wagner W. Osteonecrosis of the jaw related to sunitinib. Oral and Maxillofacial Surgery. 2011;**15**:63-66. DOI: 10.1007/s10006-010-0224-y

[49] Nicolatou-Galitis O, Migkou M, Psyrri A, Bamias A, Pectasides D, Economopoulos T, et al. Gingival bleeding and jaw bone necrosis in patients with metastatic renal cell carcinoma receiving sunitinib: Report of 2 cases with clinical implications. Oral Surgery, Oral Medicine, Oral Pathology, Oral Radiology. 2012;**113**:234-238. DOI: 10.1016/j.tripleo.2011.08.024

[50] McLeod NM, Brennan PA, Ruggiero SL. Bisphosphonate osteonecrosis of the jaw: A historical and contemporary review. The Surgeon. 2012;**10**:36-42. DOI: 10.1016/j.surge.2011.09.002

[51] Otto S, Schreyer C, Hafner S, Mast G, Ehrenfeld M, Stürzenbaum S, et al. Bisphosphonate-related osteonecrosis of the jaws—Characteristics, risk factors, clinical features, localization and impact on oncological treatment. Journal of Cranio-Maxillo-Facial Surgery. 2012;**40**:303-309. DOI: 10.1016/j.jcms.2011.05.003

[52] Fantasia JE. Bisphosphonates—What the dentist needs to know: Practical considerations. Journal of Oral and Maxillofacial Surgery. 2009;**67**: 53-60. DOI: 10.1016/j.joms.2009.01.011

[53] Bianchi SD, Scoletta M, Cassione FB, Migliaretti G, Mozzati M. Computerized tomographic findings in bisphosphonate-associated osteonecrosis of the jaw in patients with cancer. Oral Surgery, Oral Medicine, Oral Pathology, Oral Radiology, and Endodontics. 2007;**104**:249-258. DOI: 10.1016/j.tripleo.2007.01.040

[54] O'Ryan FS, Khoury S, Liao W, Han MM, Hui RL, Baer D, et al. Intravenous bisphosphonate-related osteonecrosis of the jaw: Bone scintigraphy as an early indicator. Journal of Oral and Maxillofacial Surgery.

2009;**67**:1363-1372. DOI: 10.1016/j.joms.2009.03.005

[55] Thomas C, Spanidis M, Engel C, Roos FC, Frees S, Neisius A, et al. Bone scintigraphy predicts bisphosphonate-induced osteonecrosis of the jaw (BRONJ) in patients with metastatic castration-resistant prostate cancer (mCRPC). Clinical Oral Investigations. 2016;**20**:753-758. DOI: 10.1007/s00784-015-1563-8

[56] Carlson ER, Fleisher KE, Ruggiero SL. Metastatic cancer identified in osteonecrosis specimens of the jaws in patients receiving intravenous bisphosphonate medications. Journal of Oral and Maxillofacial Surgery. 2013;**71**:2077-2086. DOI: 10.1016/j.joms.2013.05.014

[57] Ulmner M, Jarnbring F, Törring O. Osteonecrosis of the jaw in Sweden associated with the oral use of bisphosphonate. Journal of Oral and Maxillofacial Surgery. 2014;**72**:76-82. DOI: 10.1016/j.joms.2013.06.221

[58] Dodson TB. The frequency of medication-related osteonecrosis of the jaw and its associated risk factors. Oral and Maxillofacial Surgery Clinics of North America. 2015;**27**:509-516. DOI: 10.1016/j.coms.2015.06.003

[59] Gnant M, Mlineritsch B, Stoeger H, Luschin-Ebengreuth G, Knauer M, Moik M, et al. Zoledronic acid combined with adjuvant endocrine therapy of tamoxifen versus anastrozol plus ovarian function suppression in premenopausal early breast cancer: final analysis of the Austrian Breast and Colorectal Cancer Study Group Trial 12. Annals of Oncology. 2015;**26**:313-320. DOI: 10.1093/annonc/mdu544

[60] Chiang PH, Wang HC, Lai YL, Chen SC, Yen-Hwa W, Kok CK, et al. Zoledronic acid treatment for cancerous bone metastases: A phase IV study in Taiwan. Journal of Cancer Research and Therapeutics. 2013;**9**:653-659. DOI: 10.4103/0973-1482.126471

[61] Qi WX, Tang LN, He AN, Yao Y, Shen Z. Risk of osteonecrosis of the jaw in cancer patients receiving denosumab: A meta-analysis of seven randomized controlled trials. International Journal of Clinical Oncology. 2014;**19**:403-410. DOI: 10.1007/s10147-013-0561-6

[62] Stopeck AT, Lipton A, Body JJ, Steger GG, Tonkin K, de Boer RH, et al. Denosumab compared with zoledronic acid for the treatment of bone metastases in patients with advanced breast cancer: A randomized, double-blind study. Journal of Clinical Oncology. 2010;**28**:5132-5139. DOI: 10.1200/JCO.2010.29.7101

[63] Pimolbutr K, Porter S, Fedele S. Osteonecrosis of the jaw associated with antiangiogenics in antiresorptive-naïve patient: A comprehensive review of the literature. BioMed Research International. 2018;**2018**:8071579. DOI: 10.1155/2018/8071579

[64] Grbic JT, Black DM, Lyles KW, Reid DM, Orwoll E, McClung M, et al. The incidence of osteonecrosis of the jaw in patients receiving 5 milligrams of zoledronic acid: Data from the health outcomes and reduced incidence with zoledronic acid once yearly clinical trials program. Journal of the American Dental Association (1939). 2010;**141**:1365-1370

[65] Papapoulos S, Chapurlat R, Libanati C, Brandi ML, Brown JP, Czerwiński E, et al. Five years of denosumab exposure in women with postmenopausal osteoporosis: Results from the first two years of the FREEDOM extension. Journal of Bone and Mineral Research. 2012;**27**:694-701. DOI: 10.1002/jbmr.1479

[66] Bone HG, Chapurlat R, Brandi ML, Brown JP, Czerwinski E, Krieg MA, et al. The effect of three or six years of

denosumab exposure in women with postmenopausal osteoporosis: Results from the FREEDOM extension. The Journal of Clinical Endocrinology and Metabolism. 2013;**98**:4483-4492. DOI: 10.1210/jc.2013-1597

[67] Henry D, Vadhan-Raj S, Hirsh V, von Moos R, Hungria V, Costa L, et al. Delaying skeletal-related events in a randomized phase 3 study of denosumab versus zoledronic acid in patients with advanced cancer: An analysis of data from patients with solid tumors. Supportive Care in Cancer. 2014;**22**:679-687. DOI: 10.1007/s00520-013-2022-1

[68] Benford HL, Frith JC, Auriola S, Mönkkönen J, Rogers MJ. Farnesol and geranylgeraniol prevent activation of caspases by aminobisphosphonates: Biochemical evidence for two distinct pharmacological classes of bisphosphonate drugs. Molecular Pharmacology. 1999;**56**:131-140

[69] Vahtsevanos K, Kyrgidis A, Verrou E, Katodritou E, Triaridis S, Andreadis CG, et al. Longitudinal cohort study of risk factors in cancer patients of bisphosphonate-related osteonecrosis of the jaw. Journal of Clinical Oncology. 2009;**27**:5356-5362. DOI: 10.1200/JCO.2009.21.9584

[70] Kyrgidis A, Vahtsevanos K, Koloutsos G, Andreadis C, Boukovinas I, Teleioudis Z, et al. Bisphosphonate-related osteonecrosis of the jaws: A case-control study of risk factors in breast cancer patients. Journal of Clinical Oncology. 2008;**26**(28):4634-4638. DOI: 10.1200/JCO.2008.16.2768

[71] R1 K, Need A, Hughes T, Goss A. Clinical investigation of C-terminal cross-linking telopeptide test in prevention and management of bisphosphonate-associated osteonecrosis of the jaws. Journal of Oral and Maxillofacial Surgery. 2009 Jun;**67**(6):1167-1173. DOI: 10.1016/j.joms.2009.02.004

[72] Gaudin E, Seidel L, Bacevic M, Rompen E, Lambert F. Occurrence and risk indicators of medication-related osteonecrosis of the jaw after dental extraction: A systematic review and meta-analysis. Journal of Clinical Periodontology. 2015;**42**:922-932. DOI: 10.1111/jcpe.12455

[73] Yamazaki T, Yamori M, Ishizaki T, Asai K, Goto K, Takahashi K, et al. Increased incidence of osteonecrosis of the jaw after tooth extraction in patients treated with bisphosphonates: A cohort study. International Journal of Oral and Maxillofacial Surgery. 2012;**41**(11):1397-1403. DOI: 10.1016/j.ijom.2012.06.020

[74] Mozzati M, Arata V, Gallesio G. Tooth extraction in patients on zoledronic acid therapy. Oral Oncology. 2012;**48**(9):817-821. DOI: 10.1016/j.oraloncology.2012.03.009

[75] Tsao C, Darby I, Ebeling PR, Walsh K, O'Brien-Simpson N, Reynolds E, et al. Oral health risk factors for bisphosphonate-associated jaw osteonecrosis. Oral and Maxillofacial Surgery. 2013;**71**:1360-1366. DOI: 10.1016/j.joms.2013.02.016

[76] Campisi G, Fedele S, Fusco V, Pizzo G, Di Fede O, Bedogni A. Epidemiology, clinical manifestations, risk reduction and treatment strategies of jaw osteonecrosis in cancer patients exposed to antiresorptive agents. Future Oncology. 2014;**10**:257-275. DOI: 10.2217/fon.13.211

[77] Brown JJ, Ramalingam L, Zacharin MR. Bisphosphonate-associated osteonecrosis of the jaw: Does it occur in children? Clinical Endocrinology. 2008;**68**:863-867. DOI: 10.1111/j.1365-2265.2008.03189.x

[78] Hennedige AA, Jayasinghe J, Khajeh J, Macfarlane TV. Systematic review on the incidence of bisphosphonate related osteonecrosis of the jaw in children diagnosed with osteogenesis imperfecta.

Journal of Oral & Maxillofacial Research. 2014;**4**:e1. DOI: 10.5037/jomr.2013.4401

[79] Di Fede O, Panzarella V, Mauceri R, Fusco V, Bedogni A, Lo Muzio L, et al. The dental management of patients at risk of medication-related osteonecrosis of the jaw: New paradigm of primary prevention. BioMed Research International. 2018;**2018**:2684924. DOI: 10.1155/2018/2684924

[80] Abed HH, Al-Sahafi EN. The role of dental care providers in the management of patients prescribed bisphosphonates: Brief clinical guidance. General Dentistry. 2018;**66**:18-24

[81] Williams WB, O'Ryan F. Management of medication-related osteonecrosis of the jaw. Oral and Maxillofacial Surgery Clinics of North America. 2015;**27**:517-525. DOI: 10.1016/j.coms.2015.06.007

[82] Taguchi A, Shiraki M, Sugimoto T, Ohta H, Soen S, Japan Osteoporosis Society. Lack of cooperation between physicians and dentists during osteoporosis treatment may increase fractures and osteonecrosis of the jaw. Current Medical Research and Opinion. 2016;**32**:1261-1268. DOI: 10.1185/03007995.2016.1170005

[83] Yoo JY, Park YD, Kwon YD, Kim DY, Ohe JY. Survey of Korean dentists on the awareness on bisphosphonate-related osteonecrosis of the jaws. Journal of Investigative and Clinical Dentistry. 2010;**1**:90-95. DOI: 10.1111/j.2041-1626.2010.00024.x

[84] Yoneda T, Hagino H, Sugimoto T, Ohta H, Takahashi S, Soen S, et al. Antiresorptive agent-related osteonecrosis of the jaw: Position Paper 2017 of the Japanese Allied Committee on osteonecrosis of the jaw. Journal of Bone and Mineral Metabolism. 2017;**35**:6-19. DOI: 10.1007/s00774-016-0810-7

[85] Fedele S Porter SR, D'Aiuto F, Aljohani S, Vescovi P, Manfredi M, Arduino PG, et al. Nonexposed variant of bisphosphonate-associated osteonecrosis of the jaw: A case series. The American Journal of Medicine. 2010;**123**:1060-1064. DOI: 10.1016/j.amjmed.2010.04.033

[86] Del Fabbro M, Gallesio G, Mozzati M. Autologous platelet concentrates for bisphosphonate-related osteonecrosis of the jaw treatment and prevention. A systematic review of the literature. European Journal of Cancer. 2015;**51**: 62-74. DOI: 10.1016/j.ejca.2014.10.015

[87] Angiero F, Sannino C, Borloni R, Crippa R, Benedicenti S, Romanos GE. Osteonecrosis of the jaws caused by bisphosphonates: Evaluation of a new therapeutic approach using the Er:YAG laser. Lasers in Medical Science. 2009;**24**:849-856. DOI: 10.1007/s10103-009-0654-7

[88] Rupel K, Ottaviani G, Gobbo M, Contardo L, Tirelli G, Vescovi P, et al. A systematic review of therapeutical approaches in bisphosphonates-related osteonecrosis of the jaw (BRONJ). Oral Oncology. 2014;**50**:1049-1057. DOI: 10.1016/j.oraloncology.2014.08.016

[89] Freiberger JJ, Padilla-Burgos R, McGraw T, Suliman HB, Kraft KH, Stolp BW, et al. What is the role of hyperbaric oxygen in the management of bisphosphonate-related osteonecrosis of the jaw: A randomized controlled trial of hyperbaric oxygen as an adjunct to surgery and antibiotics. Journal of Oral and Maxillofacial Surgery. 2012;**70**:1573-1583. DOI: 10.1016/j.joms.2012.04.001

[90] Freiberger JJ. Utility of hyperbaric oxygen in treatment of bisphosphonate-related osteonecrosis of the jaws. Journal of Oral and Maxillofacial Surgery. 2009;**67**:96-106. DOI: 10.1016/j.joms.2008.12.003

Chapter 6

Nasal Cavity Hemangiomas

Ahmet Baki

Abstract

Hemangiomas are benign tumors originating from vascular structures in the body. Although it is common in the head and neck region, it is rarely seen in the nasal cavity and paranasal sinuses. Histologically, there are three types of hemangiomas including capillary, cavernous, and mixed types, the most common being a cavernous hemangioma. Cavernous hemangiomas in the nasal cavity usually originate from the lateral nasal wall and cause symptoms such as nasal congestion and nosebleeds.

Keywords: hemangioma, nasal septum, paranasal sinus

1. Introduction

Vascular lesions in the head and neck region originate from blood vessels or lymphatics [1].

While the terminology used to describe vascular lesions was related to the clinical appearance of the lesions rather than their physiopathological development, the first distinction that formed the basis of today's classification was made by Mulliken and Glowacki in 1982 according to the clinical and histochemical findings and cell types [2].

Nasal hemangioma was first described by Poncet and Dor in 1897 as human botryomycosis. More than half of the hemangioma affects the head and neck region, rarely the nasopharynx. Therefore it is safe to presume that hemangioma in the nasal region is a rare disease [3].

2. Hemangiomas

Hemangiomas are common, benign endothelial lesions of the skin and mucous membranes. Hemangiomas have capillary, cavernous, mixed, and hypertrophic subtypes. Capillary hemangioma is the most common subtype and is mostly seen on anterior septal cartilage. Capillary hemangioma is seen mostly in the first years of life and may show spontaneous regression (**Figure 1**) [4, 6].

Cavernous hemangioma is seen mostly in adulthood, and traumatic etiology is present. Cavernous hemangioma is rare and seen in the bone septum or lateral nasal wall. On macroscopic examination, hemangiomas can be observed to have a polypoid, smooth surface and a lobed pattern, whereas in the microscopic examination, it consists of capillaries covered with flat epithelium separated by collagen stroma. Cavernous hemangioma shows large proliferation of thin-walled blood vessels of various sizes covered with endothelium, while the mixed endothelial vascular areas form the large endothelium. These pathologies do not always differentiate from other forms of inflammatory pseudotumor (**Figure 2**) [5, 6].

Cavernous hemangiomas are uncommon in the paranasal sinuses and nose. It has been defined to originate from the inferior turbinate, vomer, lamina perpendicularis, and sinus maxillaris. Nasal mucosal hemangiomas ought to be distinguished from hemangiomas that originate from the maxilla or nasal bones which are primary osseous lesions, of which the symptoms and surgical approach are entirely different [7–12].

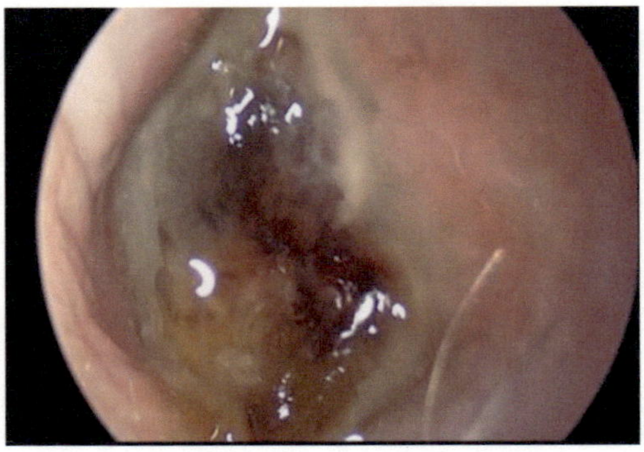

Figure 1.
Capillary Hemangioma of the Nasal Septum [5].

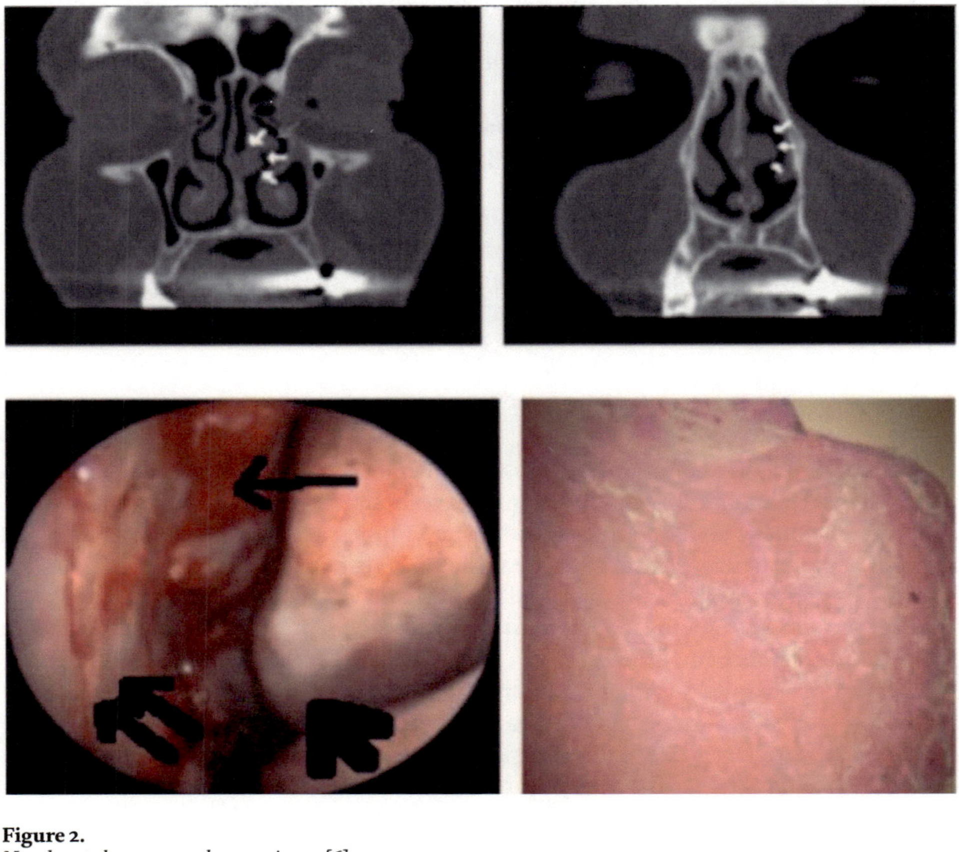

Figure 2.
Nasal septal cavernous hemangioma [6].

Although nasal hemangiomas common in the head and neck region, it is uncommonly seen in the nasal mucosa. In the nasal cavity, the most common cause is the septum and the lateral nasal wall [13].

Although nasal hemangiomas commonly affect the anterior septum as described in prior literature, nasal hemangioma has also been reported in other nasal sites such as middle turbinates, inferior turbinates, posterior part of the septum, and vestibule [14].

The most common symptom in hemangiomas located in the nasal cavity is nose bleeding; also other rare visible symptoms are nasal obstruction, runny nose, and epiphora [15]. Epistaxis and unilateral nasal obstruction were the most common presenting symptoms, followed by other nasal symptoms such as rhinorrhea. Epistaxis is the most common symptom, as demonstrated by previously published studies. In addition, extra nasal symptoms, such as facial pain and headache, are much less common [16].

In differential diagnosis, lymphangioma, venous hemangioma, angiofibroma, hemangioendothelioma, glomus tumor, and malignant nasal cavity tumors, metastatic malignancies, Wegener granulomatosis, angiofibroma, and sinonasal papilloma should be kept in mind [3, 17].

The diagnosis of cavernous hemangioma can be made based on the patient's history and clinical features of the lesion. Cavernous hemangiomas are tumors composed of vascular ectasia. They can be placed deeper in the skin, and mucous membranes additionally can involve deeper structures such as subcutaneous tissue, muscle, and bone. Hemangiomas may be localized in an area or may be common. All midline lesions such as subcutaneous cavernous hemangioma, nasal gliomas, meningocele or meningoencephaloceles, teratomas, sebaceous cysts, dermoid cysts, and fibromas, which have atypical clinical features in the nasal dorsum, should be differentiated [18].

Imaging tests such as ultrasonography (USG), computed tomography (CT), or magnetic resonance imaging (MRI) are needed to confirm vascular pathology and to demonstrate venous, arterial, or lymphatic components and whether deeper structures are involved. CT can be performed to exclude bone erosion or possible malignant transformations.

According to some authors, MRI is more effective in evaluating the connection with soft tissue and intracranial. Also, there is no radiation exposure. MRI is the first diagnostic tool that should be used for screening in patients with midline nasal mass. Negative results on imaging studies, even with contrast, do not exclude the intracranial communication. Phlebitis is typical for cavernous hemangiomas. Hypointense on T1-weighted images on MRI and hyperintense on T2 indicate the absence of coagulated blood [14, 19–22].

According to their histopathological appearance, it is possible to examine them as cavernous and capillary hemangiomas. They generally occur on the skin, and on the mucosal surfaces of the body, capillary hemangioma is a capillary ball that is located close to each other, separated by a connective tissue stroma [23]. Cavernous hemangiomas should be treated because they will never undergo involution [24].

3. Conclusion

Hemangiomas should be treated because they have the potential to cause bleeding problems and complications such as infection in the head and neck, especially in the face, ear, and nose. Agents such as steroids, interferon, and vincristine may be used in the medical treatment of hemangiomas. The use of these agents is limited due to the large number of serious toxic side effects. Propranolol, which is a nonselective beta blocker, was first introduced by Leaute-Lebeze, and it has been reported that it can be used safely in many later studies [25, 26].

Surgical excision is the treatment of choice for the treatment of nasal hemangiomas. Various surgical methods can be employed for this lesion such as excisional surgery, laser ablation, cryotherapy, and electrocoagulation. Surgical excision is a key for confirmation via histological examination and should be and remains the mode of choice of treatment for nasal hemangiomas. Surgical operation of cavernous hemangioma depends on the nature and localization of the lesion, but it should not cause functional and esthetic problems. All the patients can be successfully treated with adequate endoscopic surgical excision from the site of origin and no complications. Endoscopic resection of midline nasal tumors without intracranial extension can be performed because external approaches cause postoperative esthetic problems. Tumor resection can be removed endoscopically, leaving a safe margin. Endoscopic technique provides better esthetic results. Sclerotherapy and laser are commonly used treatment modalities. Embolization with super-selective arteriography can be used in cases with arterial component or arteriovenous fistula [14, 18, 24].

Midline elliptical incision has good functional outcomes and maintains the nasal contours, although the surgical technique for these lesion outcomes marked a scar on the midline. Treated with inferior rhinotomy and achieved excellent results [27, 28].

Lesions in the nasal type region are easily accessible after incision where transcolumellar and alarm rim incisions are combined, but it is difficult to reach larger and more complex lesions because the incision does not extend cranially [29]. A central wedge excision with vertical closure, removing excess skin, leads to a marked scar on the tip of the nose and columella, and as a result, it is recommended to avoid this wedge excision if possible [30].

Open rhinoplasty approach, and put forward that the extra skin will not be removed but rather left in place to let for contraction, which may take many months. In this approach, the excess skin remaining after the treatment of hemangioma can be considered as a disadvantage [31].

Author details

Ahmet Baki
Otorhinolaryngology Clinic, Uskudar State Hospital, Istanbul, Turkey

*Address all correspondence to: dr.ahmet170@gmail.com

References

[1] Puttgen KB, Pearl M, Tekes A, Mitchell SE. Update on pediatric extracranial vascular anomalies of the head and neck. Child's Nervous System. 2010;**26**(10):1417-1433

[2] Mulliken JB, Glowacki J. Hemangiomas and vascular malformations in infants and children: A classification based on endothelial characteristics. Plastic and Reconstructive Surgery. 1982;**69**:412-422

[3] Chi TH, Yuan CH, Chien ST. Lobular capillary hemangioma of the nasal cavity: A retrospective study of 15 cases in Taiwan. Balkan Medical Journal. 2014;**31**(1):69-71. DOI: 10.5152/balkanmedj.2014.13178

[4] Journal of Medical Case Reports. Elmer Press Inc. ISSN: 1923-4155 print, 1923-4163 online, Open Access; Journal website: http://www.journalmc.org

[5] Journal of Craniofacial Surgery. Mar 2018;**29**(2):e135-e136. DOI: 10.1097/SCS.0000000000004220

[6] Kodama S, Yoshida K, Nomi N, Fujita K, Suzuki M. Successful treatment of nasal septum hemangioma with the harmonic scalpel: A case report. Auris, Nasus, Larynx. 2006;**33**(4):475-478

[7] Kim HJ, Kim JH, Kim JH, Hwang EG. Bone erosion caused by sinonasal cavernous hemangioma: CT findings in two patients. American Journal of Neuroradiology. 1995;**16**:1176-1178

[8] Hayden RE, Luna M, Goepfert H. Hemangiomas of the sphenoid sinus. Otolaryngology and Head and Neck Surgery. 1980;**88**:136-138

[9] Nakahira M, Kishimoto S, Miura T, Saito H. Intraosseous hemangioma of the vomer: A case report. American Journal of Rhinology. 1997;**11**:473-477

[10] Graumüller S, Terpe H, Hingst V, Dommerich S, Pau HW. Intraossäres Hämangiom der Lamina perpendicularis ossis ethmoidalis. HNO. 2003;**5**:142-145

[11] Engels T, Schörner W, Felix R, Witt H, Jahnke V, Kavernöses Hämangiom d. Sinus maxillaris. HNO. 1990;**38**:342-344

[12] Osborn DA. Hemangiomas of the nose. The Journal of Laryngology and Otology. 1959;**73**:174-179

[13] Çaylakli F, Çagici AC, Hürcan C, Bal N, Kizilkiliç O, Kiroglu FMD. Cavernous hemangioma of the middle turbinate: A case report. Ear, Nose, & Throat Journal. 2008;**87**(7):391-393

[14] Puxeddu R, Berlucchi M, Ledda GP, Parodo G, Farina D, Nicolai P. Lobular capillary hemangioma of the nasal cavity: A retrospective study on 40 patients. American Journal of Rhinology. 2006;**20**(4):480-484

[15] Işılay D, Fuat B. Nazal Septumda Pyojenik Granülom: Olgu Sunumu. Acıbadem Üniversitesi Sağlık Bilimleri Dergisi. 2011;**2**(1):8

[16] Fasunla AJ, Adebola OS, Okolo CA, Adeosun AA. Nasal septal lobular capillary haemangioma in West Africa sub-region: A case report. Cases Journal. 2009;**8, 2**:8952

[17] Batsakis JG. Tumors of the head and neck. In: Clinical and Pathological Considerations. 2nd ed. Baltimore, MD: Williams & Wilkins; 1979. pp. 291-312

[18] Harley EH. Pediatric congenital nasal masses. Ear, Nose, & Throat Journal. 1991;**70**:28-32

[19] Reilly JR, Koopman CF, Cotton R. Nasal mass in a pediatric patient. Head & Neck. 1992;**14**:415-418

[20] Lusk RP, Lee PC. Magnetic resonance imaging of congenital midline nasal masses. Otolaryngology and Head and Neck Surgery. 1986;**95** (3 Pt 1):303-306

[21] Barkovich AJ, Vandermarck P, Edwards MS, Cogen PH. Congenital nasal masses: CT and MR imaging features in 16 cases. AJNR. American Journal of Neuroradiology. 1991;**12**:105-116

[22] Itoh K, Nishimura K, Togashi K, Fujisawa I, Nakano Y, Itoh H, et al. RM imaging of cavernous hemangioma of face and neck. Journal of Computer Assisted Tomography. 1986;**10**:831-835

[23] Chawla OP, Oswal VH. Hemangiopericytoma of the nose and paranasal sinuses. The Journal of Laryngology and Otology. 1987;**101**:729-737

[24] Yokoyama M, Inouye N, Mizuno F. Endoscopic management of nasal glioma in infancy. International Journal of Pediatric Otorhinolaryngology. 1999;**51**:51-54

[25] Evans SE. İnfantil Hemanjiyomlar. Türk Derm. 2011;**45**:133-137

[26] Hsu TC, Wang JD, Chen CH, Chang TK, Wang TM, Chou CM, et al. Treatment with propranolol for infantile hemangioma in 13 Taiwanese newborns and young infants. Pediatrics and Neonatology. 2012;**53**:125-132

[27] Pitanguy I, Machado BH, Radwanski HN, Amorim NF. Surgical treatment of hemangiomas of the nose. Annals of Plastic Surgery. 1996;**36**(6):586-592

[28] Demiri EC, Pelissier P, Genin-Etcheberry T, Tsakoniatis N, Martin D, Baudet J. Treatment of facial haemangiomas. British Journal of Plastic Surgery. 2001;**54**(8):665-674

[29] Faguer K, Dompmartin A, Labbé D, Barrellier MT, Leroy D, Theron J. Early surgical treatment of Cyrano-nose haemangiomas with Rethi incision. British Journal of Plastic Surgery. 2002;**55**(6):498-503

[30] Mc Carthy JG, Borud LJ, Schreiber JS.Hemangiomas of the nasal tip. Plastic and Reconstructive Surgery. 2002;**109**(1):31-40

[31] Jackson IT, Sosa J. Excision of nasal tip hemangioma via open rhinoplasty: A skin-sparing technique. European Journal of Plastic Surgery. 1998;**21**:265-268

Chapter 7

Structural and Functional Disorders of the Temporomandibular Joint (Internal Disorders)

Nedeljka Ivkovic and Maja Racic

Abstract

There are many factors that can cause damage to the temporomandibular joint (TMJ) structures or impair normal functional relationships between condyle, disc and eminence. The main symptoms associated with TMJ dysfunction are pain, limited mobility of the mandible, spasticity of the masticatory muscles and sound that is produced in the joint during mandibular movement. Pain originates from nociceptors located in soft tissue of the joint. If the soft tissue structures are not in inflammation, the pain is sharp, sudden and intense tightly connected to the movements in the TMJ. If the inflammation is presented, the pain is constant and increases with the movements in the joint. TMJ dysfunction is manifested by feeling stiffness of the joint, limited and/or altered opening of the mouth with deviation or deflection of the mandible. Individual or multiple sound produced by the TMJ are most often the consequence of the disturbed function of the condyle-disc complex, the morphological incompatibility of the joint surfaces or degenerative changes in them. The signs and symptoms of disease and dysfunction of TMJ are different and depend on the duration of the disorders and its chronicity as well as on the individual sensitivity of the patients. Proper identification of symptoms and precise diagnosis are therefore essential for future treatment.

Keywords: TMJ, internal disorders, signs, symptoms, therapy

1. Introduction

Temporomandibular joint (TMJ) is susceptible to various diseases affecting other synovial joints. Due to its position it is exposed to trauma, and its functional link with the occlusal complex which makes it very sensitive to any occlusal disorders. Any force that overloads the TMJ complex can cause damage to the joint structures or disrupt the normal functional relationship between condyle, disc and articular eminence, resulting in dysfunction or pain, or both. Systemic joint disorders may also affect TMJ.

Diseases and functional disorders of the TMJ can be globally divided into several categories:

- deviations in the form of articular surfaces,

- disorders in the functions of the condyle-disc complex,

- inflammatory diseases of the TMJ,
- degenerative TMJ disorders,
- ankylosis of TMJ.

This classification is based on the recommendations of the American Academy of Orofacial Pain 1993 [1].

The basic symptoms that accompany the diseases and dysfunction of TMJ are: pain, abnormal jaw movement, spasm of masticatory muscles and joint sounds produced by the joints during mandibular movements [2].

a. The pain that origins from any joints including the TMJ, is called arthralgia.

   Arthralgia is triggered by receptors located in the soft tissue of the joint. Such receptors (nociceptors) contain discal ligaments, retrodiscal tissue and articular capsule. Arthralgia from the soft-tissue structures of the non-inflammatory joint represents a sharp, sudden and intense pain that is closely related to the joint movements. If, however, the inflammation of the soft-tissue structures of the affected joint has occurred, the pain will be constant and increase during mandibular movements. Course of pain can be acute or chronic [2].

b. Disturbed joint function is a common accompaniment to all joint disorders. TMJ dysfunction can occur in various forms but their major effects are the limitations and/or alterations of jaw movements. This is manifested by the feeling the stiffness of the joint, limited mouth opening with deviation or deflection of the mandible on the affected side and limited movement to the contralateral side [2, 3].

c. The sound signals produced by the joint are the most common consequence of the dysfunction of the condyle-disc complex, the morphological incompatibility of articular surfaces and their degenerative changes. The sound signals produced by the joint may occur as individual short-duration sounds at opening or when opening and closing the mouth, referred to as clicking ("click") or as multiple, rough and scratched sounds, which are called as "crepitation" [2, 3].

2. Deviations in the form of articular joint surfaces

2.1 Defects on the articular joint surfaces

The most common defects on the articular joint surfaces occur in the upper joint compartment and affect the articular eminence or the upper surface of the disc, thus preventing normal translatory movements.

Causes. Irregularities of articular joint surfaces may arise as a result of trauma (e.g., a blow to the lower jaw in open mouth), or are the result of inflammatory processes in the joint, structural or development anomalies [2, 4].

Signs and symptoms. These disorders are usually not accompanied by pain. Opening or closing the mouth is difficult and limited due to the existence of mechanical obstructions on the articular joint surfaces. Due to an attempt to overcome an obstruction, the mandibular deviation to the affected side is observed in the opening of the mouth, which is directly related to the barrier position in the translatory cycle. As the obstacle is located at a certain location, the mandibular deviation always appears at the same opening or closing point.

Deviation can be followed by clear single sound—"click", followed by normal opening or closing of the mouth. The click always occurs at the same level of opening or closing motion and should be distinguished from the reciprocal click in patients with disc displacement with reduction. In the disc displacement with reduction click is rarely heard at the same level of opening or closing the mouth [2, 4, 5].

Therapy. Patients education is very important in managed of these symptoms. Patients with defects on the articular joint surfaces should learn how to move the jaw to avoid the obstacle. Chewing predominantly to the side of the defect may be helpful in reducing intracapsular pressure in the affected joint. Stabilization splint recommended during the night and 1–2 hours during the day for at least 8–10 weeks, can reduce the pressure on the joint structure and the muscular hyperactivity, but does not usually remove the sounds. If dysfunction is significant and if pain occurs, the possibility of surgical therapy should be considered [2, 4, 5].

2.2 Thinning of articular disc and perforation of disc

Causes. Excessive and long-term load of the joint under the conditions of the closed mouth and the dental contacts may result in the thinning of the central zone of the disc. The constant excessive pressure in that zone can lead to perforation of the disc [2, 6, 7].

Signs and symptoms. The symptoms depend on the size of the defect and changes in the disc or articular surface of the condyle. In cases of perforated disc, movements in the joint were accompanied by characteristic crunching or cracking sounds (crepitations). Pain is usually an early companion of these disorders, but over time, as the defect increases, it may decrease or completely disappear. Joint sensitivity and muscle spasms most likely complement the clinical findings, and pain is related to mandibular movements. Disc thinning and perforation are difficult to diagnose clinically [5]. Diagnosis is best placed with some of the appropriate radiological methods, such as arthrography, arthroscopy, or magnetic resonance images (MRI) [8–10].

Therapy. If the joint and surrounding muscles are sensitive or painful to palpation, it is recommended to wear a stabilization splint during the night and 1–2 hours during the day for at least 8–10 weeks, that will reduce the joint load, muscular spasm and possible pain. If using medications is considered for pain reduction, it is recommended to use NSAID naproxen (Naprosyn) 500 mg two times per day minimum of 3 weeks [11]. As it is not possible to regenerate the disc, in cases of mandibular movements accompanied by permanent intensive pain, surgery is recommended [5].

3. Function disorders of condyle-disc complex

3.1 Disc derangements (mechanism of disorder)

These disorders are series of dysfunction that are most often the result of previous diseases, trauma, or occlusal disharmony. Disorders are caused by changes in the relationship between condyle and disc and the disturbance of their functional activity. In the normal joint the disc is bound to the medial and lateral condyle pole by discal ligaments. Therefore translational movement in the healthy joint is possible only between the condyle-disc complex and the articular eminence. The only physiological movement between condyle and disc is rotation. The amount of rotation of the disc in normal circumstances depends on the shape of the disc, the degree of interarticular pressure and the synergic function of the upper head of the lateral pterygoid muscle and the upper layer of the bilaminar zone [2, 10, 12–16].

In opening the mouth and moving the condyle-disk complex forward, the upper layer of the bilaminar zone is tensed and retracted (rotates) the disc in the posterior direction. The interarticular pressure increasing during the mouth opening maintained the condyle below the thin intermediate zone of the disc and prevented the thicker anterior disc border from being pulled between the condyle and eminence.

The upper layer of the bilaminar zone is the only structure that can pull the disc backwards. This force only works when the condyle is moved forward and it extends and tightens the upper layer of the bilaminar zone. There is no tension in the retrodiscal tissue during the closing of mouth. The disc rotates forward thanks to the function of the upper head of the lateral pterygoid muscle, when the mouth closing. This muscle part is activated and pulls the disc forward, while the condyle-disc complex slides back and up. The moderate rotation of the disc, which occurs in the normal joint under the mechanisms described, allows the disc and condyle to remain in intimate contact during all movements and all mandibular positions. In the healthy joint, the articular surfaces of the condyle, disc, and eminence are smooth and sliding, which ensures unobtrusive movements without any friction. The normal relationship between condyle and disc in mandibular movements is also maintained due to the specific form of disc.

The biconcave form of the disc and its thickening borders itself ensures the stability of the disc condition while the interarticular pressure increases during the opening of the mouth also helps to center the disc on the condyle. Medial and lateral discal ligaments support the maintenance of disc because they avoid any translatory movement between condyle and disc [2, 10, 12–16].

If, however, the form of the disc is changed and the discal ligament is elongated, the translatory movement between the condyle and the disc becomes possible. The amount of this movement depends on the change in the form of disc and the degree of elongation of discal ligament. Discal ligaments are not elastic and after elongation they retain that length.

Under the closed mouth, interarticular pressure is very low. If the disc ligaments are stretched, the disc can move on the articular surface of the condyle. Since in the closed mouths the upper layer of the bilaminar zone has no influence on the position of the disc, the tone of the upper head of the lateral pterygoid muscle may influence the disc to assume the anterior position on the condyle. Moving the disk forward is medially limited by the length of the discal ligaments and the thickness of the posterior disc border. If this condition lasts longer, the posterior disc border can be thinned, making it easier for its antero-medial dislocation. In such cases, the articular surface of the condyle no longer rests below the intermediate zone of the disc during closing mouths, but under its thinned posterior disc border or, even in the retrodiscal tissue.

This condition is referred to as a functional derangement of the disc and is initially difficult to register. Later, there is a pain, usually associated with chewing. If the anterior displacement of the disc is more pronounced, the joint function may be compromised. During the mouth opening, the condyle moves forward, a short translatory movement between the condyle and the disc is performed first, ensuring that the condyle takes its normal position below the intermediate zone of the disc. This relation of condyle and disc is then maintained during the further opening of the mouth under the action of interarticular pressure which increases at the opening of the mouth.

During the closing of the mouth the fibers of the retrodiscal tissue actively assist in restoring the condyle to the normal position, which it occupies when the mouth is opened. The interarticular pressure maintains intimate contact between the condyle and the disc during the translational closing movement and does not allow the anterior, thicken disc border thread between the condyle and the articular eminence. However, when the closing movement is complete, the interarticular pressure decreases and the tension in the retrodiscal tissue is reduced, the tone in the upper head of the lateral pterygoid muscle will have an effect on the anterior displacement of the disc [2, 10, 12–16].

The basic characteristic of this functional disorder is the presence of translational motion between the condyle and the disc at the beginning of the opening and at the end of the mouth closure, which does not exist in the normal joint. During this pathologic translation, increased interarticular pressure or deformed articular disc may prevent undisturbed crossing of articular surfaces. This raises the sudden, distorted movement of the condyle that skips the barrier to take normal position below the intermediate zone of the disc. This sudden skip of the condyle motion usually accompanies a characteristic sound, which is referred to as a "click" at the mouth opening. After this sound, normal relation between condyle and disc is established during further movement of the opening.

This condyle-disc interact is presented during mouth closing all the way till the very end. However, when the mouth is closed and the interarticular pressure decreased, the disc is again displaced forward (and medially) under the tone of the upper head of the lateral pterygoid muscle.

If the displacement is small this shift is usually not followed by a characteristic sound. A single "click" at the mouth opening indicates an early stage of dysfunction.

If the condition is prolonged, the dysfunction is increased. Continuously anteriorly displaced disc leads to permanent elongation of the discal ligaments, including the lower layer of the retrodiscal tissue. The posterior disc border continues to thinning, and the condyle lies practically on the retrodiscal tissue when the mouth closed. Morphological changes in the disc in the area where the condyle is now positioned may cause a secondary "click" in the final stages of closing the mouth just before the condyle takes the final position. Disc is most often moved forward, or anteromedial, but it also appeared the medial, lateral and even posterior displacement of the disc. Displacements of the articular disc represent a series of pathological conditions that progressively worsen over time. These conditions usually begin with disc displacement with reduction, which is usually not accompanied by pain or major function disorders. In some patients, this condition aggravates, takes a heavier form of dysfunction, disc displacement without reduction, while in others the level of the displacement of the disc is prolonged for long time (**Figure 1**). The reason for these differences is not always clear. The presence of various factors that may contribute to the development of dysfunction, such as loss of lateral teeth, systemic stability of the ligaments or the presence of parafunctional activities, has certainly a significant influence. In diagnosing disc displacement, clinical examination is not always sufficient to determine the actual condition, especially in cases where dysfunction does not cause greater discomfort. Special X-ray techniques, such as arthrography or MRI, are often needed to confirm a clinical diagnosis. However, it must be emphasized that the painless joint with mild mouth signaling is not an indication of the use of complicated and expensive X-ray methods. The clinician must determine whether arthrography or MRI is crucial for determining the correct treatment [8–10].

3.1.1 Disc displacement with reduction

In this disorder when the mouth is closed, disc does not take a normal position between condyle and articular eminence, but is displaced forward, or forward and medial, and during opening of the mouth it returns to approximately normal position on the condyle [2, 10, 12–17]. In some cases, this may be accompanied by increased muscular activity, pain, and limitation of mandibular movements.

Causes. The most common cause is trauma. Macrotrauma such as blow to the jaw or microtrauma associated with orthopedic instability and muscle hyperactivity.

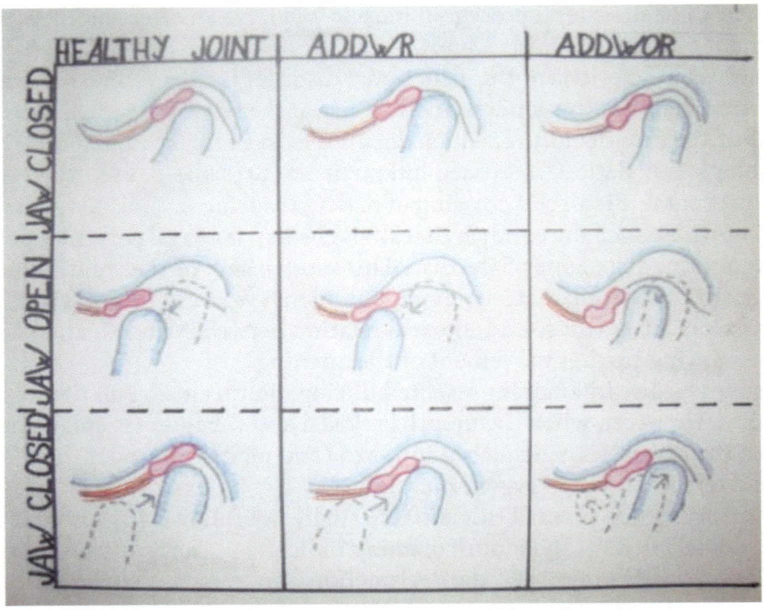

Figure 1.
The position of TMJ disc during mouth opening and closing in three different conditions: healthy joint, anterior disc displacement with reduction (ADDWR) and anterior disc displacement without reduction (ADDWOR).

Signs and symptoms. The characteristic signs of the disc displacement with reduction is clear individual sound (like skipping through an obstacle) during the opening of the mouth, or when opening and closing the mouth. This sound which is referred to as a "click" can be heard at any point in the translatory cycle, and it occurs when the condyle passes through the posterior disc border in order to lie beneath its intermediate zone. During the closing of the mouth it is also possible to detect a softer "click" resulting from the disc being returned to the displaced anterior position. This dual audible signal at the opening and at the end of the mouth closure is marked as a "reciprocal click" [5, 10, 12–17].

The following clinical sign that can be easily detected in these patients is the deviation of the middle line of the mandible to the affected joint at the earliest stage of mouth opening. This is because of the temporary blockade of condyle translation caused by disc displacement. When the disc takes a normal position in relation to the condyle, during mouth opening, the translational movement forward and down as well as the middle line of the mandible return to normal. The deviation from the deflection of the mandible should be distinguished. Deviation is the initial turning of the mandible to the affected joint due to a temporary obstacle. The mandible returns to the central position when the obstacle passes (**Figure 2**). In the deflection, the middle line of the mandible moves from the beginning to the end of the movement of the opening to the affected side and does not return to the center (**Figure 3**).

Pain is not always a companion to the anterior disc displacement. If present, it is usually stimulated by tensed disc ligaments or it is caused by the condyle pressure on the retrodiscal tissue.

The amount of mandibular movements in this disorder is usually normal and in fact the diameter of the maximum opening of the mouth may be greater than normal. Limited opening of the mouth, if present, is the most common consequence of muscular spasm caused by pain, rather than mechanical obstruction of the articular disc [5, 10, 12–17].

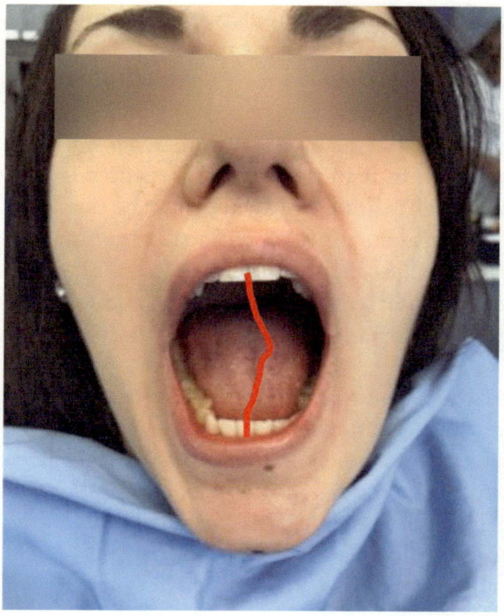

Figure 2.
Mandibular deviation during mouth opening associated with disc displacement with reduction.

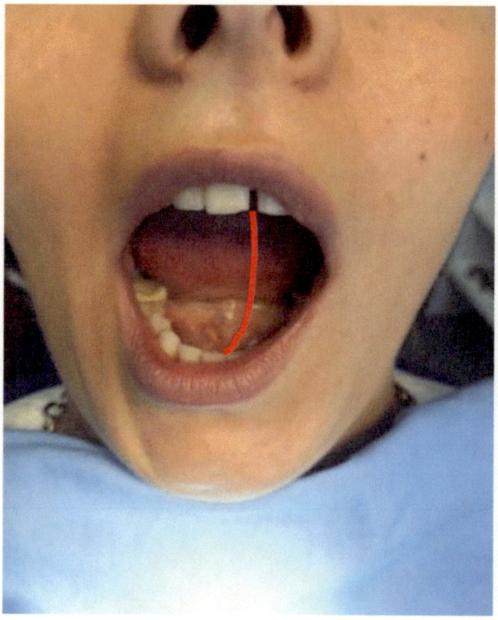

Figure 3.
Mandibular deflection during mouth opening associated with disc displacement without reduction (affected right side).

Therapy. All cases of anterior disc displacement with reduction do not require treatment. Anterior disc displacement with reduction may persist for years without progression because of physiological adaptation of the TMJ structure. In many cases elongation of the retrodiscal fibers occurs, which then functions as a modified extension of the posterior disc border. In other words, modified retrodiscal tissue accepts the condyle load. If the patient does not complain of pain or significant damage to the joint function (limited mouth opening) and the surrounding muscles are not sensitive to palpation, no therapy is required. These patients should, of course, be monitored and periodically monitored in order to detect possible progression of the disease.

Sensitivity of the joint to palpation in patients with single or reciprocal click, even in the absence of pain, indicates that there was no adaptation of the joint tissue to this condition. The patient should be aware that the dysfunction has a progressive course and that painful sensations may also occur, especially when it comes to patient with parafunctions [16–18].

If the disc displacement with reduction is accompanied by pain, all management measures should be taken to alleviate or eliminate pain and second to improve function.

The benefit of the use of some intraoral devices in the management of patients with disc displacement with reduction is still subject of discussion. Most commonly applied intraoral devices are repositioning splint and stabilization splint [18–23]. Recently in the literature, the modified mandibular splint has been mentioned, which achieves significant success rate in eliminating joint sounds and patients had no complications because of occlusal changes [24].

The basic aim of the repositioning therapy is to temporarily stabilize the mandible in an appropriate anterior position that allows the disc, if possible, to take a normal position on the condyle, and that the retrodiscal tissue releases the pressure and thus eliminates the pain and clicking sounds of the joint. Much more important is moving the condyle forward, which should enable the adaptive and regenerative processes in the retrodiscal tissue. Why this adaptation occurs in some patients, and in others not, it is not yet clarified. The goal of repositioning therapy is, therefore, to eliminate pain and allow relaxation and regeneration, actually transformation of the retrodiscal tissue [10, 18–20, 22, 23] (**Figures 4–6**).

Repositioning therapy may, however, also have some consequences. Therefore, repositioning therapy can be considered as a temporary treatment that reduces pain and joint sounds in a relatively short period of time. The results of long-term use of the repositioned splint are, however, not encouraging, especially in terms of eliminating the sound signals. In spite of these shortcomings, repositioning therapy has its place within the noninvasive (conservative) methods of treating patients with anterior disc displacement with reduction [18–20, 22, 23].

Some authors recommend that treatment begins by introducing a stabilization splint during a certain time because adverse long-term effects are minimized. A

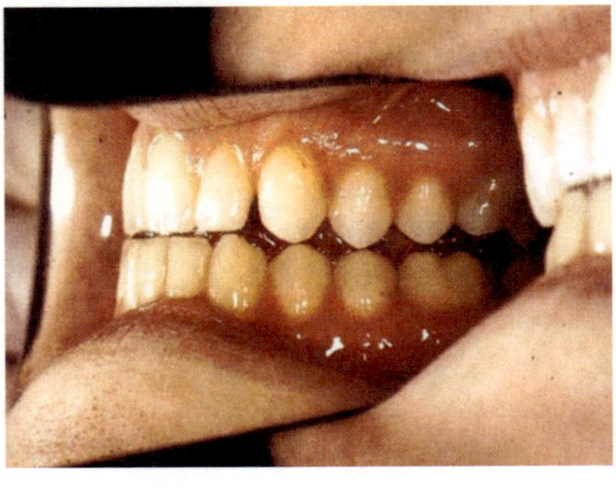

Figure 4.
Mandibular protrusion position, about 2–3 mm in front of the maximal intercuspal position, the reciprocal sounds are unheard in patient with disc displacement with reduction.

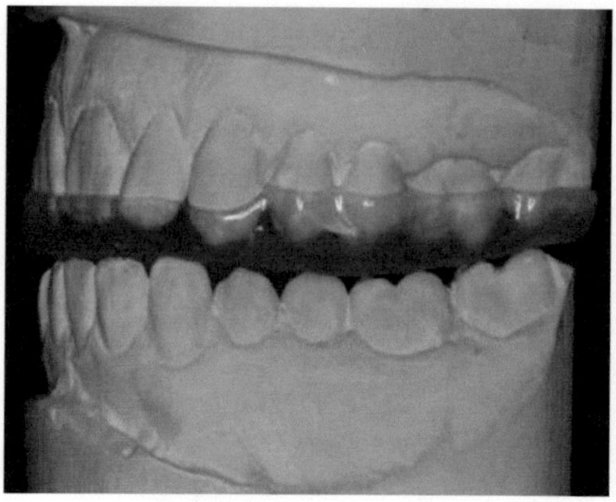

Figure 5.
Stone cast model with repositioning splint (contact position).

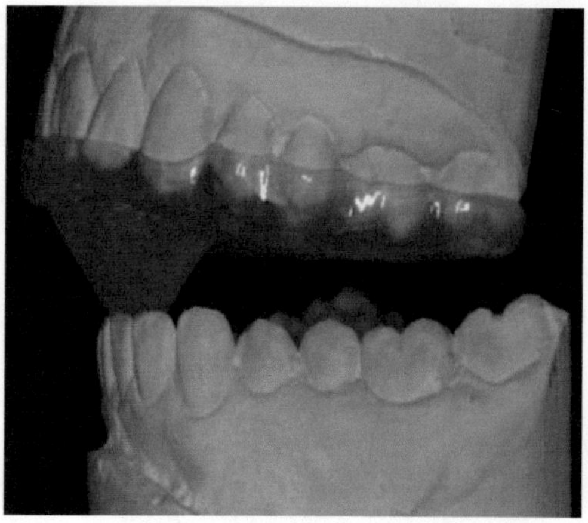

Figure 6.
Stone cast model with repositioning splint.

stabilization splint is applied in the upper jaw at night and, preferably, 1–2 hours during the day for several weeks (**Figures 7** and **8**). If there is no symptom reduction during stabilization splinting therapy, repositioning therapy should be continued. Before performing a repositioning splint, it is good to perform a test that will show whether the mandibular repositioning eliminates the sounds and the amount of propulsion required. This is done by maximizing the mouth opening in order to reduce the disc to a normal position. At the upper dental arch, place several layers of wax for the shaping, then the mandible is easily brought to the protrusion position, about 2–3 mm in front of the maximal intercuspal position. If the sounds are heard when reaching the mandible in that position, it is unlikely that the repositioning therapy will be successful in correcting the condyle-disc relationship. Clicking in the early (initial) mouth opening phase has a better prognosis than clicking at later stages. It indicates a minor disorder, a smaller amount of disc displacement, and less damage to the discal ligaments.

After 2–3 months of application the repositioning splint worn 24 hours a day including when the patient is eating (if possible), if the pain is significantly reduced or eliminated, the anterior repositioning splint should be reconverted to the stabilization splint. Treatment is considered successful if the patient does not have any pain, regardless of whether the joint sounds are present. If pain occurs again, the treatment with anterior reposition of mandible should be repeated. However, before

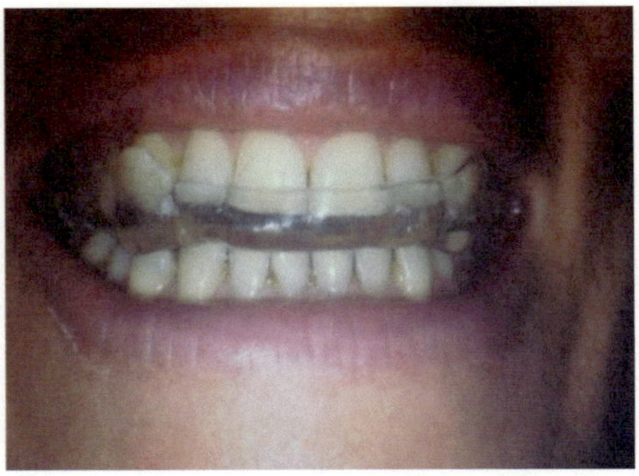

Figure 7.
Stabilization splint in patient with disc displacement with reduction.

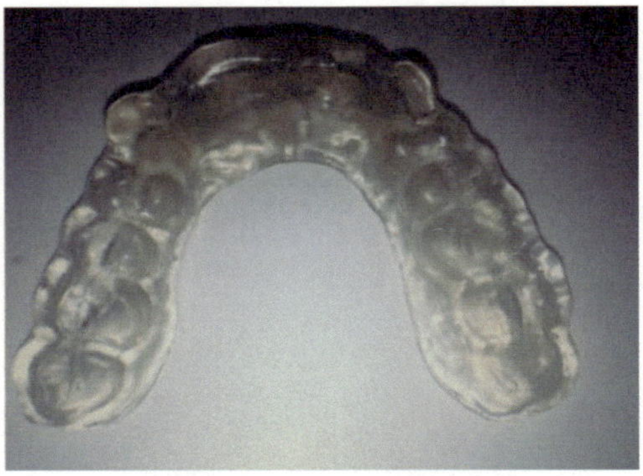

Figure 8.
Fabricated stabilization splint.

recreating the repositioning splint, it is necessary to check whether there are additional factors that jeopardize treatment (bruxism, harmful habits) and whether the patient wears a splint as instructed by the physician. Certainly, the patient should be warned of the need for maximum control of parafunctional activities, eliminating bad habits, avoiding strong and long-lasting chewing, hard food, etc. [12, 20, 22, 23].

Disc displacement with reduction sometimes requires immediate treatment, even though the patient does not complain on pain. In patients with intermittent joint blockades, treatment should begin immediately, as such conditions can lead to serious injuries to the joint, most often the disc displacement without reduction. All pain-related disc displacements require treatment.

3.1.2 Disc displacement without reduction

This condition is characterized by anterior or antero-medial disc displacement in closed mouth conditions, where the disc does not return to the normal condyle relationship during mouth opening or condyle translation. Translational movements of the condyle are limited or disabled as it cannot pass under the dislocated and deformed disc. Pressed disc changes its shape, from biconcave to biconvex, and the anterior disc connection is relaxed. The contact between the condyle, the disc, and the articular eminence is lost, the space which normally occupies the disc is reduced, and the deformed disc is below the condyle. This results in restricted translation of the condyle in the affected joint, limited opening of the mouth, and sometimes with complete blockade of the mouth opening ("closed lock").

Causes. Except of cases where this occurred immediately after some trauma, anterior disc displacement without reduction was a consequence of the gradual, progressive degeneration of the joint structure preceded by symptoms of anterior disc displacement with reduction [5, 12].

Due to more efficient approach to therapy and overall prognosis, the state of anterior disc displacement without reduction can be divided into two stages—acute and chronic.

3.1.2.1 Acute disc displacement without reduction

Signs and symptoms. The most prominent clinical sign of acute disc displacement without reduction is very limited mouth opening, maximum about 25–30 mm (**Figures 9** and **10**). When opening the middle line of the mandible, it suddenly turns to the affected side. The protrusion of the mandible is also limited and associated with the deflection of the mandible on the affected side. Since the displaced disc represents a mechanical barrier for each translatory motion of the condyle, the lateral movement of the mandible to the opposite side is also limited. However, for differential diagnosis it is important that the lateral movement of the mandible to the affected side is not limited and that it takes place within normal range. The lateral movement restriction on the affected side may, however, occur later because of pressure of the condyle on inflamed retrodiscal tissue, not due to mechanic obstruction. This situation is characteristic for disc displacement without reduction resulting in trauma. Acute disc displacement without reduction, due to the accompanying inflammation of the capsule, retrodiscal connective tissue and the discal ligaments, is always followed by pain. The activity of master and temporalis muscles on the affected side is also disturbed. The spasm of these muscles increases the pain and still limits the opening of the mouth. Acute condition has no sounds, as its function is practically blocked, but when the disc displacement becomes chronic, degenerative changes may occur on the articular surfaces of the joints causing the characteristic crepitations.

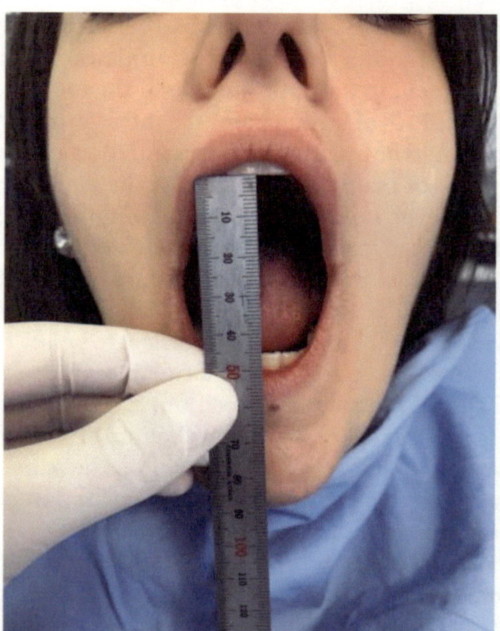

Figure 9.
Normal range of mouth opening in healthy person.

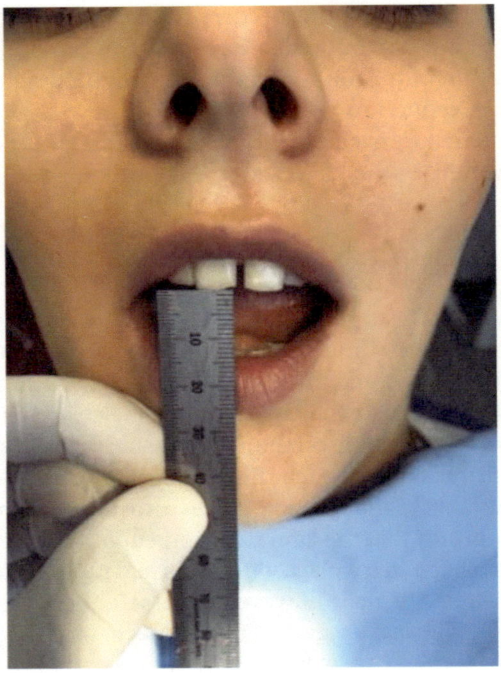

Figure 10.
Limited mouth opening in patient with disc displacement without reduction.

Since limited mouth opening can be the result of muscular spasm, differential diagnosis should determine the true cause of this occurrence. It is known that contraction of the mandibular elevator muscles may limit vertical movements of mandible but does not significantly affect the lateral and protrusive range of motion. On the contrary, the intracapsular cause of mandibular movement restraints, such as disc displacement without reduction, leads to obstruction of all translational motion of the condyle in the affected joint and thus to the limitation of mouth opening, propulsion and lateral movement to the opposite side. If the movements of the mandible are not limited by the presence of strong pain, the intracapsular cause of mandibular obstruction usually permits the opening of the mouth by a pure rotation range of 25 mm. In cases of spasms or painful contraction of the mandibular elevator muscles, mouth opening may, however, be limited to several millimeters [5, 12, 25, 26].

Therapy. In the acute stage, the initial therapy is directed to repositioning the dislocated disc by manual mobilization. This procedure should allow the separation of the condyle from the articular eminence by manual traction (pulling the mandible downwards), to provide space for returning the dislocated disc. To do this, the upper layer of the bilaminar zone must be healthy and functionally capable of retracting the disc backwards [25–27]. Prior to manual reposition, it is good to start with medication combination such as anxiolytic agent diazepam (Valium) 2.5 mg four times per day for 1 week than 5 mg four times per day for 2 weeks to alter the patient's reaction to the stress and NSAID Ibuprofen 600 mg four times per day for 3 weeks that will reduce pain and inflammation. If a secondary muscle spasm is present, it is good to prescribe some muscular relaxation cyclobenzaprine (Flexeril) 10 mg every night [11].

The manual rearrangement therapist performs it by pressing the thumb to the lower teeth or the lower alveolar ridge of the affected side pulling the lower jaw downwards and separating the condyle from the articular eminence, thus providing a space for restoring the disc. If the reposition succeeds, as it can be seen from the considerably increased range of mouth opening, propulsion, and movement on the contralateral side, immediate repositioning splint should be introduced to prevent disc re-displacement. This splint should be made in advance and now modified so as to stabilize the mandible in the propulsive position 2–3 mm in front of the maximal intercuspal position. The patient needs to carry a splint constantly during the day and night, even during the meal, for the first 2–4 days before beginning only night-time use for at least 10 days. Also, a diet with only soft food should be prescribed. The patient should report at least once a week to evaluate the condition and eventually adjust the splint. If the disc is in the optimal position after this period, the repositioning splint can be replaced by a stabilization splint. If the joint blockade is repeated in spite of applied therapy, it is necessary to reanalyze the degree of dysfunction (the amount of disc displacement, possibility of its restoration) in order to establish a definitive therapy plan. The frequency of temporary joint blockades or long period disc displacement without reduction significantly reduces the chance for successful treatment (reposition) due to irreversible changes in joint tissue. Single, sudden joint blockade accompanied by limited mouth opening and intense pain has a much better prognosis, especially if the blockade is a consequence of a sudden trauma that has affected a healthy joint. The patient should be advised to use soft food and to maximally reduce the range of mandibular movements. If the attempt of manual reposition of the disc displacement fails, other alternatives should be considered [5, 12, 25–27].

The diagnosis of the dislocated disc is also confirmed by some radiographic methods that allow the analysis of soft tissue of the joint (arthrography, MRI) [8–10].

3.1.2.2 Chronic disc displacement without reduction

In patients with chronic disc displacement without reduction, the disc is deformed and its last attachment is non-functional, so returning it to normal position is impossible.

Signs and symptoms. The pain, if it exists, is not of such intensity as in acute cases. Auscultation can be used to detect crepitations due of the mandibular movement, indicating the presence of degenerative changes in the joints. Patients with chronic disc displacement without reduction often report data on the progressive course of the dysfunction, the sounds produced by the mouth opening, and the occasional blockades of the joint followed by limited mouth opening and pain. Exceptions are patients in whom this condition is caused by trauma [25, 26].

Therapy. The procedure for returning the disc to normal position by manual mandibular mobilization is indicated if this condition does not last too long. In most patients with chronic disc displacement without reduction, manual mandibular mobilization does not provide satisfactory results. In such cases, a decision on possible therapeutic procedures should be made. One possibility is to introduce stabilization splint therapy during the night and, preferably, 1–2 hours during the day for 8–10 weeks regardless of the position of the disc that will allow the transformation and adaptation of the retrodiscal tissue and the other alternative is surgical therapy. The decision basically depends on the pain intensity that follows the dysfunction. It is advisable not to undertake surgical intervention if it is possible to try different types of reversible occlusal therapy, e.g., with a stabilization splint, which will stimulate regeneration and transformation of the retrodiscal tissue. Transformation and adaptation of the retrodiscal tissue to increased loads in some patients passes painless while others are accompanied by painful symptoms and limited joint function. Certain systemic or local factors such as episodes of bruxism, poor oral habits, and emotional stress may contribute to this condition. The existence of such alterations is best determined by arthrography, arthroscopy or MRI [8–10]. If the pain cannot be eliminated by the conservative therapy and the movements of the mandible are very limited, surgery is indicated [10, 15, 25, 26].

3.2 Joint hypermobility (subluxation)

This disorder was previously referred to as "subluxation".

Pathogenesis. During the normal mouth opening while the condyle-disc complex moves forward along the articular eminence, the disc performs a rotational motion on the head of the condyle directed backwards. If the opening of the mouth continues beyond the normal limits of the translatory cycle of the condyle-disc complex, the further posterior rotation of the disc can be disabled and further opening of the mouth occurs without rotation of the disc. This can cause the condyle to skip the top of the articular eminence, with a characteristic sound, and put itself in front of it [4, 5, 28, 29].

Causes. Hypermobility is most commonly caused by the inherited weakness of the discal ligaments. This condition, however, can appear after intubation for general analgesia, after long-lasting dental interventions at lateral teeth or may be the result of sudden trauma. The diameter of mandibular motion during yawning or taking food in some people is also habitually higher than the average. The joint hypermobility is often associated with too steep articular eminence, which is common in patients with skeletal class II [30, 31].

Usually both joints are included, but hypermobility may be unilateral if it is the result of the joint hypomobility of the opposite side.

Signs and symptoms. Immediately in front of the end of the mouth opening, there is a short delay in the movement of the condyle, after which they skip the top of the articular eminence and move forward and upward. Initially, this movement was irregular and accompanied by a characteristic joint sounds. Hypermobility is usually not accompanied by pain if the condition does not become chronic. In differential diagnosis, joint hypermobility which is usually accompanied by extreme opening of the mouth and characteristic sounds (skip), should be distinguished from the joint "click" at the opening of the mouth which indicates the disc displacement with reduction. The sound created by the joint hypermobility is heard at the time of the maximum opening of the mouth [4, 5, 28, 29].

Therapy. It is very important to educate patient regarding the cause and movement that create the interference. A large number of patients can reduce and control this disorder by simply reducing the mouth opening range. They are used to taking smaller snacks, limiting mouth opening or supporting the mandible during yawning or visiting a dentist. Exercises that strengthen the elevator of mandible can also reduce the joint hypermobility [4, 5, 28, 29]. If hypermobility is accompanied by pain, arthroscopic surgery is recommended [32].

When the hypermobility of TMJs is part of the general (systemic) hypermobility of all the joint structures, it can be considered benign and no intervention should be undertaken [28, 29]. However, the joint hypermobility can lead to more difficult conditions, such as recurrent mandibular dislocation.

3.3 Spontaneous dislocation

In the literature, it is referred as a mouth closure or "open lock"" [2, 33, 34].

Pathogenesis. This disorder is characterized by the inability of the patient to spontaneously close his mouth after an excessive opening and it is the result of a blockade of condyle under the articular eminence. This usually happens in patients with a longer history of joint hypermobility, but it can also occur spontaneously after a strong yawning or mouth open for a long time.

Causes. Dislocation arises due to the excessive and irregular movement of the condyle in front of the articular eminence and the subsequent spasm of the mandibular elevators.

Signs and symptoms. The mandible is blocked in the opened mouth position and the patient is anxious because of the inability to close the mouth. This can be followed by a pain that is most commonly due to mandibular elevators spasms and overstretched discal ligaments. There is acute malocclusion with contacts only on the last molars and with open bites in the front. Condyles are in the anterior position compared to the articular eminence, and in some patients there is clearly the presence of depression in the preauricular area previously filled with condylas" [2, 4, 5].

Therapy. Patients with dislocation of the condyle-disc complex are terribly frightened and often have strong pains. That it why they need to approach them very gently and encouragingly. Any attempt to coarse or violently mouth closure should be avoided because it can enhance the spasm of elevators. The patient should be advised to calm down and relax if possible, and then open his mouth as much as possible to relax the mandibular elevator (the effect of reciprocal inhibition). By placing the thumb of one and the other hand behind the molar and energizing the pressure first downwards, and then back until the patient opens his mouth as much as he can, the doctor tries to return the blocked mandible. In some cases, it is recommended to give an injection with a solution of a muscular relaxant or to give mandibular anesthesia.

If manual repositioning fails in the attempt, it is recommended to trigger the vomiting reflex by touching the soft palate by mirror. This inhibits the activity of the elevators and increases the chances of its manual repositioning. If the dislocation of the condyle-disc complex often repeats (becoming a chronic phenomenon), it is best to train the patient how to bring the mandible back to normal position using exercises like joint hypermobility [2, 33, 34].

Surgical intervention can be undertaken if this condition is often repeated and accompanied by pain. It usually consists of eminectomy (reduction of peak articular eminence) or eminoplasty (a surgical increase in inclination of the articular eminence) to prevent subsequent dislocations [35, 36].

4. Inflammatory and degenerative diseases of the temporomandibular joint

4.1 Inflammatory diseases in TMJs

Depending on the tissue in which the process takes place, inflammation of the TMJ is referred to as capsulitis, synovitis and retrodiscitis.

Pathogenesis. Excessive damage to the TMJ which comes because of parafunctions, trauma or infection may cause an inflammatory response in the fibrous capsule, the synovial membrane or the retrodiscal tissue. Continuous pain, sometimes while resting, which increases during function, is the main symptom of inflammatory processes in the TMJ. As soon as the inflammation calms down, the pain stops. In addition to continuous pain, a secondary central excitatory effect, such as muscle spasm, hyperalgesia (excessive sensitivity to external stimuli), allodynia (a painful reaction to light stimuli of the affected area), often follow inflammatory processes in the TMJ [37].

4.1.1 Capsulitis and synovitis

Capsulitis (inflammation of the external fibrotic layer of the joint capsule) and synovitis (inflammation of the synovial membrane) have almost the same clinical picture and are considered to be a unique clinical entity.

Causes. These inflammatory processes can occur secondary as a result of trauma or after sudden and excessive stretching of the capsular and discal ligaments.

Long-term keeping of mouth open during dental interventions can also cause these processes. Capsulitis and synovitis are often associated with internal disorders in the TMJ, such as disc displacement, hypermobility or dislocation of the mandible [36–39].

Signs and symptoms. Pain during the resting which increases during the function or after load is the main symptoms of capsulitis and synovitis. The mandibular mobility is limited. The lateral polar region of the condyle is susceptible to palpation, and the mild swelling area is often noticeable. Generally there are no changes in the bone structure of the joint when observed radiographically. Magnetic resonance imaging can provide information on the presence of inflammatory edema of some joint tissue. Laboratory analyzes show the presence of inflammatory process [11, 37–39].

Therapy. Therapy depends largely on the etiology of an inflammatory process. If macrotrauma initiates the process, NSAID naproxen (Naprosyn) 500 mg two times per day for minimum of 3 weeks [11], ultrasound therapy are provided, with advice on maximum control and reduction of the mandibular movement, wet warm meals with soft, almost liquid nutrition. In cases where the patient is relieved, cold pack is used for pain and swelling reduction. It may be applied three or four times a day for 10–20 minutes. To make a cold pack, put ice cubes in a plastic bag, wrap the bag in a clean, thin towel or cloth. Never put ice or a cold pack directly on the skin.

In the case of acute persistent pain, injection of corticosteroids (methylprednisolone 5–20 mg with 0.5 ml local anesthetic using 23–27 gauge, 05–1 inch needle) into the joint or joint area can reduce the pain and the inflammation. It should be cautious with corticosteroids because of the potential for damage to joint tissue. It is not recommended to administer more than three injections at short intervals [11]. Corticosteroids should not be given if acute purulent infection is present.

If the inflammation is a consequence of chronic, repeated microtrauma or it has been secondary due to disc displacement, specific therapy is used to remove the source of the microtrauma or to allow the replacement of the dislocated disc [11, 37–39]. The use of stabilization splint for several weeks during the night, in these cases, reduces bruxism, reduces pressure on the joint and eliminates muscular spasm. Reposition splint therapy can help in cases where the primary cause is anterior disc displacement. This therapy minimizes the trauma of the discal ligaments.

4.1.2 Retrodiscitis

Condyle pressure on richly vascularized retrodiscal tissue with a lot of nerves located behind an articular disc can lead to inflammation and swelling with significant functional disturbances.

Causes. Retrodiscitis may be caused by a sudden blow in the chin which suppresses condyle to the retrodiscal tissue. It may also be the result of chronic microtrauma caused by a non-physiological position of the condyle in people with anterior disc displacement. [11, 37–41].

Signs and symptoms. The main symptoms are the continuous pain and sensitivity of the lateral and posterior region of TMJ to palpation. Pain increases when teeth are in occlusion or when the mandible is moved to the affected side, or whenever condyle presses the retrodiscal tissue. If the swelling is presented, the condyle can be moved anteriorly, resulting in acute loss of contact between the lateral teeth on the affected side [41]. Since chewing on the opposite side can increase pressure and cause pain, the patient should be advised to chew on the affected side.

Therapy. If retrodiscitis is a consequence of sudden trauma, the treatment is the same as for capsulitis or synovitis. It is recommended to use NSAID naproxen (Naprosyn) 500 mg two times per day for minimum of 3 weeks [11]. The patient is advised to limit mandibular movement, soft, almost liquid nutrition, and various forms of physical therapy are most often used in the treatment. The initiation of stabilizing splint reduces the load of retrodiscal tissue and promotes its recovery. If retrodiscitis is caused by anterior disc displacement, the application of the repositioning splint is indicated. In cases of severe pain, corticosteroids can be moderately used. The therapy primarily aims to eliminate inflammation and then to normalize the function of the joint [5, 11, 40, 41].

4.2 Arthritides

Degenerative diseases of the TMJ differ significantly from those that have been written since they primarily damage bony articular surfaces of condyle and fossa. Some classifications characterize these diseases commonly referred to as arthritides [42]. The different types are: osteoarthritis, osteoarthrosis, polyarthritides.

Degenerative diseases of the joint systems may be of local character, then they only affect specific joint structures such as TMJ or may, however, be part of the general systemic disease of all joints in the body (polyarthritis).

Pathogenesis. The articular surfaces of the TMJ have great potential for adaptation to numerous functional procedures. During the course of life, progressive remodeling processes of articular surfaces maintain a constant balance between shape and function. However, if the joint structures are permanently exposed to excessive non-physiological damage, the repairing abilities of the joint tissue can be overcome, and then the articular surfaces of the joints lose the ability to adapt to an increased load and become softened followed by resorption of subarticular bone. This can lead to permanent damage to the articular surfaces of the joint over time. The problem of maintenance of homeostasis can also occur under normal TM load in cases where the defensive abilities of the body and total adaptive capacity are weakened due to aging or numerous systemic disorders [42–46].

4.2.1 Osteoarthritis of the TMJ

Osteoarthritis is one of the most common arthritides affecting the TMJ. Osteoarthritis usually develops gradually and is limited in character. Degenerative processes in the TMJ even without a certain therapy end in about 3 years. The pain is reduced and the joint function somewhat regenerates, the volume of mandibular movements increases, and the creptions become less expressive. However, structural changes in the bone components of the joint are definitive. This stabilized condition is sometimes referred to as osteoarthrosis after the inflammatory process retreated and when pain is no longer present [11, 37, 39, 40, 42–46].

Causes. It is related to the secondary inflammation of the synovial joint membrane and is therefore accompanied by pain. In some patients, the inflammatory process develops as a result of overload of the joint for reasons that are not fully clarified.

Signs and symptoms. The main symptom of osteoarthritis of the TMJ is constant localized pain. In the initial stage of the disease, the pain is very intense, especially during the function, and it calms down at the resting mandibular position. Later the pain is present during the rest, too. The patient wakes up with a stiff joint. When opening and closing the mouth, creptions are present. Cold and wet weather often increases the pain. Due to the pain, the mandibular mobility is limited and its turning on the affected side during mouth opening, as well as the lateral movement restriction on the opposite side are noticeable. The area of the joint is painfully sensitive to palpation, and pain occurs at each joint load. A swelling is often present in the joint area, especially if trauma is one of the etiologic factors. Myalgia and spasm of masticatory muscles usually accompany osteoarthritis of the TMJ and are part of the protective mechanism. Muscular response can also be due to CNS irritation by deep pain and inflammation of the joint [11, 12, 37, 39, 40, 42, 43].

Changes in TMJ in lateral phases of disease can be observed on radiographic images, especially on the articular surfaces of the condyle in the form of the flattened surface, the presence of osteophytes, the cystic formation in the subchondral bone and the reduction of the joint space [12, 44].

Therapy. Initially therapy should be focused on treating the patient about the behavior in the acute phase of the disease. The course of the disease is of limited character (self- limiting) and the various models of therapy are mainly focused on the reduction of pain and the stimulation of the repair processes.

The patient needs to take soft, almost fluid food; to avoid any function during the painful stages of the disease. Antirheumatics, NSAID, naproxen (Naprosyn) 500 mg two times per day for minimum of 3 weeks [11] or combination anxiolytic agent diazepam (Valium) 2.5 mg four times per day for 1 week than 5 mg four times per day for 2 weeks to and NSAID Ibuprofen 600 mg four times per day for 3 weeks are prescribed to reduce the pain and inflammation of the joints. The use of muscle relaxants cyclobenzaprine (Flexeril) 10 mg every night or sedatives clonazepam (Klonopin) 0.25 mg every night, increased by 0.25 each week to a maximum of 1 mg per day in patients with muscular spasms is suggested. Corticosteroid injections (methylprednisolone 5–20 mg with 0.5 ml local anesthetic using 23–27 gauge, 05–1 inch needle) help in cases of intense pain [11, 12, 37, 39, 40, 44]. Since mechanical overload of the joint is the main cause of osteoarthritis, it is recommended to use a stabilizing splint during the night and, preferably, 1–2 hours during the day for 6–8 weeks [12]. If the pain is unbearable, if it does not decrease after the above mentioned treatment, the possibility of surgery is considered.

4.2.2 Osteoarthrosis of the TMJ

Osteoarthrosis is a non-inflammatory degenerative process that changes the morphology of joint components and mainly affects the articular surfaces of the TMJ and the subchondral bone. When bony changes are active, the condition is called osteoarthritis. As remodeling occurs the condition can become stable, yet the bony morphology remains altered [12, 45, 46].

Pathogenesis. Fibrocartilaginous overlay loses high-elastic properties and therefore the load is transmitted directly to the subchondral bone. As the degenerative process progresses, enhanced osteoclastic activity can lead to the thinning and perforation of the articular cortex on condyle. In addition, cystic formations in the medullar areas of the subcortical bone of the condyle are developed. After the decay of the fibrocartilaginous overlay, the subchondral bone remains without cover and there is generalized erosion of the condyle surface and changes in its surface. The proliferation of bone tissue at the edges of the condyle results in the formation of osteophyte.

Causes. It is the most common consequence of the long-term non-physiological load of the joint surfaces. Repeated strong pressure on the TMJ structure results in degeneration of fibrocartilaginous tissue covering the condyles. Osteoarthrosis of TMJ may arise secondary as a consequence of disc displacement, or as the loss of the amortizing function of the articular disc. However, osteoarthrosis may also be due to mechanical overload of the joint, when it occurs before the disc displacement. Since changes in articular joint surfaces can lead to degenerative changes in the disc, in some cases disc displacement may be the result of osteoarthrosis rather than its cause [12, 45–47].

Signs and symptoms. Osteoarthrosis is characterized by the absence of painful sensitivity to joint palpitation. The mobility of the mandible is, however, limited by turning on the affected side during mouth opening. Crepitations (multiple scarring sign), caused by changes in the joint surfaces, are usually presented at the opening and closing of the mouth and are much more expressive in the late stages of the disease [12, 45–47]. In addition to the clinical examination, radiography that provides data on structural changes in the subcortical bone of the condyle confirms the diagnosis of osteoarthrosis [8–10].

Therapy. In the absence of pain, osteoarthrosis represents a stable adaptive phase, no special therapy is indicated. However, if the changes in the joint surfaces are so severe that they change the occlusal relationships, an occlusal therapy that will stabilize occlusion is desirable [12, 45–47].

4.2.3 Polyarthritis

Systemic polyarthritis can also involve the TMJ. The clinical picture is similar to that of localized osteoarthritis of TMJ.

Pathogenesis. Diseases are manifested by degenerative changes in the fibrocartilaginous cover of condyle and subchondral bone, and inflammation of the joint capsule and synovial membrane. Changes in TM joints begin on the periphery of a nonspecific inflammatory process leading to degeneration of synovial tissue. Hypertrophic synovial tissue fills the synovial spaces, disabling normal functioning of the joints, followed by pain. Enzymes released from synovial tissue lead to destruction and erosion of bone structures of condyles and temporal bone. Over time, these processes cause fibrous ankylosis of the joint followed by occlusofacial deformities.

Causes. In the category of polyarthritis, many diseases of different etiologies are included: rheumatoid arthritis, juvenile rheumatoid arthritis, psoriatic arthritis, Lyme disease, infectious arthritis, ankylosing spondylitis as well as metabolic disorders, hyperuricemia [12, 45–48]. In the case of polyarthritis, both TMJ are affected.

Signs and symptoms. The acute stage of the disease is characterized by the pain and sensitivity of the TMJ on palpation. Other inflammatory signs, such as the swelling, redness in the joint area, increased temperature and, of course, limited functions may be present. There are often crepitations. Symptoms usually occur with parafunctions, strong chewing, and sometimes during normal function. Expressed degenerative changes in condyles that accompany rheumatoid arthritis may result in displacement of the condylar attachments up and down, within the fossa articularis, resulting in acute occlusion disorders. This is manifested by a retroposition of mandible and occlusal contacts only in the area of the last molars. The radiographic finding usually indicates strong destructive changes in the bone structure of the joints, starting from irregular bone erosion to severe and complete destructions of the condyle. Flatness of articular eminence and other changes in bone structure of fossa articularis are also often present.

Therapy. Since the TMJ disorder is secondary, it is important to establish a proper diagnosis of the systemic illness and treat it. Definitive diagnosis is based on laboratory tests, anamnestic data and physical examination. If the condition of the organism as a result of general therapy improves, signs and symptoms of the TMJ diseases can also be withdrawn.

Therapy of TMJ disease in these cases is palliative. It is recommended to rest the joints, take antiflogistics, analgesics and sedatives to relieve pain. The most common recommended drugs are NSAID, naproxen (Naprosyn) 500 mg two times per day for minimum of 3 weeks [11] or combination anxiolytic agent diazepam (Valium) 2.5 mg four times per day for 1 week than 5 mg four times per day for 2 weeks to and NSAID Ibuprofen 600 mg four times per day minimum for 3 weeks. In some patients, treatment may be attempted by stabilization occlusal split during the night for several weeks, which significantly reduces muscle hyperactivity, which relieves pain. Although there is an obvious occlusion instability, the use of irreversible occlusal therapy should be considered well and, of course, do not undertake anything to relieve the underlying disease and eliminate the inflammation in TM joints.

If occlusal therapy is necessary because of the occlusion stabilization, the position of the condyle in relation to the articular eminence should be well analyzed. In cases of extreme damage of the TM joints and complete occlusion disorders, orthognathic surgery is indicated [12, 45–48].

5. Ankylosis of the TMJ

Ankylosis is defined as immobilization or concrescence of the joint structures, caused by degenerative diseases, hemarthrosis secondary to joint injuries or surgical interventions. Inability or restriction of movement in the TMJ may be caused by fibrosis or bone tissue, which is less frequent [49, 50].

5.1 Fibrosis ankylosis

Hyperplasia of the fibrous tissue in the joint can lead to the ankylosis of the condyle, disc or retrodiscal tissue for the posterior wall of the joint capsule, articular fossa or the articular eminence.

Causes. The most common cause of fibrous ankylosis of the TM joint is hematoma resulting from trauma. Ankylosis can also occur as a result of extensive synovitis, but also as a result of surgical intervention. Adhesions inside the joint can also cause fibrosis ankylosis. They are usually a result of long-term load of the joint structures, for example in people with parafunctional activities. In such situations, normal lubrication of the joint surfaces is reduced, resulting in intermittent disc adhesion on the articular eminence. In this stage, the adhesions are relatively easily removed by condyle movement (mouth opening exercises). However, if their maturation is allowed, fibrous tissue hyperplasia may occur which leads to permanent fixation of the articular surfaces. Although most of the adhesions occur in the upper joint space, between the disc and the articular eminence, the adhesion is also noticeable in the lower joint space, between the disc and the condyle, Arthroscopic finding indicates that pathological adhesions are most commonly found in the lateral third of the joint. This condition is referred to as "lateral blockade syndrome".

Fibrosis may also occupy the joint capsule (capsular fibrosis), forming the binder fibers of the fibrous tissue inside the capsule, and may also cause general capsular thickening. This condition is characterized by a painless limitation of the mandible movement on the opposite side.

Signs and symptoms. If the disc is fixed for fossa or articular eminence, there is limited translation of condyle-disc complex. Mouth opening is limited. During the opening, mandible turns to the affected side, and the lateral movements are limited on the opposite side. If there is pain, it is variable, and it is caused by tightening of discal ligaments. The limitations of the mandibular movement caused by fibrotic ankylosis should be distinguished from the restriction of motion caused by anterior disc displacement without reduction because these two conditions require different therapies. Arthroscopy, arthrography and MR that indicate the condition of soft joint tissues can greatly assist in differential diagnostics [8–10].

Therapy. Treatment depends on the presence of pain and degree of dysfunction. If the patient has a satisfying function with little discomfort, treatment is not necessary. If the condition, however, is unbearable with pain and drastic reduction of function, the choice treatment is arthroscopic surgery and subsequent physical therapy. When there is a significantly reduced opening of the mouth, the method of choice is open joint surgery, which involves removing entire fibrous tissue and primary reconstruction of the joint [49].

5.2 Bone ankylosis

Causes. This condition is caused by the proliferation of bone tissue, which results in the concrescence of the bone structure of the joint and its complete immobilization. It can be distinguished as a result of infection, fracture, or chronic inflammatory process in the joint [50].

Signs and symptoms. Clinically, the condition is very similar to fibrous ankylosis. The movements of the mandible are almost completely blocked, with the turning of chin center on the affected side when trying to open the mouth. Lateral movements on the opposite side are practically limited. Native radiography provides the best data on the size and location of the bond between the articular surfaces. Bone ankylosis, as well as fibrosis, is usually not accompanied by pain.

In a clinical finding, one-sided ankylosis is dominated by a poorer development of the affected side—the middle of the chin and the bite center are moved to that side. In the case of bilateral ankylosis, there is a so-called " bird's face" appearance. The lower jaw is generally undeveloped. Due to the inability to open the mouth, hygiene is usually poor, with a consequent set of teeth caries [50].

Therapy. Treatment depends on the condition in each case and the degree of dysfunction, as this ankylosis type is usually not followed by pain. In patients with severe dysfunction, the only treatment that can give good results is surgical removal of bone attachment and formation of new articular surfaces. Both fibrosis and bone ankylosis are most often followed by contractures of mandibular elevators, which must be taken into account within the overall therapy program [50].

6. Conclusion

The signs and symptoms of disease and dysfunction of TMJ are different in various disease groups and depend on the duration of the disease and its chronicity and as well as on the individual sensitivity of the patient. Proper identification of symptoms and precise diagnosis are therefore essential for future treatment.

Conflict of interest declaration

I confirm that there is no conflict of interest.

Author details

Nedeljka Ivkovic[1*] and Maja Racic[2]

1 Departmant of Oral Rehabilitation, Faculty of Medicine, University of East Sarajevo, Bosnia and Herzegovina

2 Departmant of Primary Health Care and Public Health, Faculty of Medicine, University of East Sarajevo, Bosnia and Herzegovina

*Address all correspondence to: neda.ivkovic3@gmail.com

References

[1] McNeill C. Temporomandibular Disorders: Guidelines for Classification, Assessment and Management. American Academy of Orofacial Pain. 2nd ed. Chicago: Quintessence Publishing Co; 1993. pp. 27-38

[2] Okeson JP. Management of Temporomandibular Disorders and Occlusion. 6th ed. St Luise: Mosby; 2008. pp. 164-216 (ch. 8)

[3] Guler N, Yatmaz PI, Ataoglu H, Emlik D, Uckan S. Temporomandibular internal derangement: Correlation of MRI findings with clinical symptoms of pain and joint sounds in patients with bruxing behavior. Dento Maxillo Facial Radiology. 2003;**32**:304-310. DOI: 10.1259/dmfr/24534480

[4] Bell WE. Temporomandibular Disorders: Classification, Diagnosis and Management. 3rd ed. Chicago: Year Book Medical; 1990. pp. 289-357

[5] Okeson JP. Management of Temporomandibular Disorders and Occlusion. 6th ed. St Luise: Mosby; 2008. pp. 404-453 (ch. 13)

[6] Kondoh T, Westesson PL, Takahashi T, Seto K. Prevalence of morphological changes in the surfaces of the temporomandibular joint disc associated with internal derangement. Journal of Oral and Maxillofacial Surgery. 1998;**56**(3):339-343

[7] Molinari F, Manicone PF, Raffaelli L, Raffaelli R, Pirronti T, Bonomo L. Temporomandibular joint soft-tissue pathology, I: Disc abnormalities. Seminars in Ultrasound, CT, and MR. 2007;**28**(3):192-204

[8] Marotti M. Imaging of temporomandibular joint disorders. Medical Science. 2010;**34**:135-148

[9] Hasan NMA, Abdelrahman TEF. MRI evaluation of TMJ internal derangement: Degree of anterior disc displacement correlated with other TMJ soft tissue and osseous abnormalities. The Egyptian Journal of Radiology and Nuclear Medicine. 2014;**45**:735-744

[10] Rathod D. Internal derangement of temporomandibular joint etiology, pathophysiology, diagnosis and management: A review of literature. International Journal of Advanced Research. 2016;**2**(7):643-649

[11] Gauer RL, Semidey MJ. Diagnosis and treatment of temporomandibular disorders. American Family Physician. 2015;**91**(6):378-386

[12] Okeson JP. Joint intracapsular disorders: Diagnostic and nonsurgical management considerations. Dental Clinics of North America. 2007;**51**(1):85-103. DOI: 10.1016/j.cden.2006.09.009

[13] Paesani D. Etiopathogenesis of TMJ disc displacements. In: Manfredini D, editor. Current Concepts of Temporpmandibular Disorders. Chicago: Quintessence Publishing Co; 2010. pp. 81-110 (ch. 5)

[14] Stegenga B, LGM DB. TMJ disc derangements. In: Laskin DM, Greene CS, Hylander WL, editors. Temporomandibular Disorders: An Evidence-Based Approach to Diagnosis and Treatment. Chicago: Quintessence Publishing Co; 2006. pp. 125-136 (ch. 8)

[15] Young AL. Internal derangements of the temporomandibular joint: A review of the anatomy, diagnosis, and management. Journal of Indian Prosthodontic Society. 2015;**15**(1):2-7. DOI: 10.4103/0972-4052.156998

[16] Manfredini D. Etiopathogenesis of disk displacement of the temporomandibular joint: A review of the mechanisms. Indian Journal of

Dental Research. 2009;**20**(2):212-221. DOI: 10.4103/0970-9290.51365

[17] Sato S, Goto S, Nasu F, Motegi K. Natural course of disc displacement with reduction of the temporomandibular joint: Changes in clinical signs and symptoms. Journal of Oral and Maxillofacial Surgery. 2003;**61**(1):32-34. DOI: 10.1053/joms.2003.50005

[18] Lalue-Sanches M, Gonzaga AR, Guimaraes AS, Ribeiro EC. Disc displacement with reduction of the temporomandibular joint: The real need for treatment. Journal of Pain and Relief. 2015;**4**(5):200. DOI: 10.4172/21670846.1000200

[19] Yuasa H, Kino K, Kubota E, Kakudo K, Sugisaki M, Nishiyama A, et al. Primary treatment of temporomandibular disorders: The Japanese society for the temporomandibular joint evidence-based clinical practice guidelines, 2nd edition. Japanese Dental Science Review. 2013;**49**(3):89-98. DOI: 10.1016/j.jdsr.2013.05.002

[20] Conti PCR, Corrêa ASM, Lauris JRP, Stuginski-Barbosa J. Management of painful temporomandibular joint clicking with different intraoral devices and counseling: A controlled study. Journal of Applied Oral Science. 2015;**23**(5):529-535. DOI: 10.1590/1678-775720140438

[21] Kuzmanovic Pficer J, Dodic S, Lazic V, Trajkovic G, Milic N, Milicic B. Occlusal stabilization splint for patients with temporomandibular disorders: Meta-analysis of short and long term effects. PLoS One. 2017;**12**(2):e0171296. DOI: 10.1371/journal.pone.0171296

[22] Clark GT, Minakuchi H. Oral appliances. In: Laskin DM, Greene CS, Hylander WL, editors. Temporomandibular Disorders: An Evidence-Based Approach to Diagnosis and Treatment. Chicago: Quintessence Publishing Co; 2006. pp. 377-390

[23] Devi J, Verma M, Gupta R. Assessment of treatment response to splint therapy and evaluation of TMJ function using joint vibration analysis in patients exhibiting TMJ disc displacement with reduction: A clinical study. Indian Journal of Dental Research. 2017;**28**(1):33-43. DOI: 10.4103/ijdr.IJDR_154_16

[24] Huang IY, Wu JH, Kao JH, Chen CM, Chen CM, Yang YH. Splint therapy for disc displacement with reduction of thetemporomandibular joint. Part I: Modified mandibular splint therapy. The Kaohsiung Journal of Medical Sciences. 2011;**27**(8):323-329. DOI: 10.1016/j.kjms.2011.03.006

[25] Yura S. Natural course of acute closed lock of the temporomandibular joint. The British Journal of Oral & Maxillofacial Surgery. 2012;**50**(7):646-649. DOI: 10.1016/j.bjoms.2011.10.014

[26] Al-Baghdadi M, Durham J, Araujo-Soares V, Robalino S, Errington L, Steele J. TMJ disc displacement without reduction management: A systematic review. Journal of Dental Research. 2014;**93**(7 Suppl):37S-51S. DOI: 10.1177/0022034514528333

[27] Yoshida H, Fukumura Y, Suzuki S, Fujita S, Kenzo O, Yoshikado R, et al. Simple manipulation therapy for temporomandibular joint internal derangement with closed lock. Asian Journal of Oral and Maxillofacial Surgery. 2005;**17**(4):256-260. DOI: 10.1016/S0915-6992(05)80021-4

[28] Hirsch C, John MT, Stang A. Associatation between generalized joint hypermobility and sings and diagnoses of temporomandibular disorders. European Journal of Oral Sciences. 2008;**116**(6):525-530. DOI: 10.1111/j.1600-0722.2008.00581.x

[29] Kavuncu V, Sahin S, Kamanli A, Karan A, Aksoy C. The role of systemic hypermobility and condylar hypermobility in temporomandibular joint dysfunction syndrome. Rheumatology International. 2006;**26**(3):257-260. DOI: 10.1007/s00296-005-0620-z

[30] Ren YF, Isberg A, Wesetessen PL. Steepness of the articular eminence in the temporomandibular joint. Oral Surgery, Oral Medicine, and Oral Pathology. 1995;**80**(3):258-266

[31] Henrikson T, Nilner M, Kurol J. Signs of temporomandibular disorders in girls receiving orthodontic treatment. A prospective and longitudinal comparison with untreated class II malocclusions and normalocclusion subjects. European Journal of Orthodontics. 2000;**22**(3):271-281

[32] devi Devaraj S, Pradeep D. Internal derangement of temporomandibular joint-a review. IOSR Journal of Dental and Medical Sciences. 2014;**13**(3):66-73

[33] Kai S, Kai H, Nakayama E, Tabata O, Tashiro H, Miyajima T, et al. Clinical symptoms of open lock position of the condyle. Relation to anterior dislocation of the temporomandibular joint. Oral Surgery, Oral Medicine, and Oral Pathology. 1992;**74**(2):143-148

[34] Nitzan DW. Temporomandibular joint "open lock" versus condylar dislocation: Signs and symptoms, imaging, treatment, and pathogenesis. Journal of Oral and Maxillofacial Surgery. 2002;**60**(5):506-511. DOI: 10.1053/joms.2002.31846

[35] Williamson RA, Mc Namara D, Mc Auliffe W. True eminectomy for internal derangement of the temporomandibular joint. The British Journal of Oral & Maxillofacial Surgery. 2000;**38**(5): 554-560. DOI: 10.1054/bjom.2000.0467

[36] Puelacher WC, Waldhart E. Miniplate eminoplasty: A new surgical treatment for TMJ dislocation. Journal of Cranio-Maxillo-Facial Surgery. 1993;**21**(4):176-178. DOI: 10.1016/S1010-5182(05)80109-X

[37] O'Connor RC, Fawthrop F, Salha R, Sidebottom AJ. Management of the temporomandibular joint in inflammatory arthritis: Involvement of surgical procedures. European Journal of Rheumatology. 2017;**4**(2):151-156. DOI: 10.5152/eurjrheum.2016.035

[38] Murakami K, Segami N, Fujimura K, Iizuka T. Correlation between pain and synovitis in patients with internal derangement of the temporomandibular joint. Journal of Oral and Maxillofacial Surgery. 1991;**49**(11):1159-1161. DOI: 10.1016/0278-2391(91)90407-D

[39] Herb K, Cho S, Stiles MA. Temporomandibular joint pain and dysfunction. Current Pain and Headache Reports. 2006;**10**(6):408-414

[40] Malik P, Rathee M, Sehrawat R. Temporomandibular disorders and their management. American Journal of Public Health Research. 2015;**3**(3-2):1-5. DOI: 10.11648/j.ajhr.s.2015030302.11

[41] Marinho LH, McLoughlin PM. Lateral open bite resulting from acute temporomandibular joint effusion. British Journal of Oral and Maxillofacial Surgery. 1994;**32**(2):127-128

[42] McNeill C. Temporomandibular Disorders: Guidelines for Classification, Assessment and Management. American Academy of Orofacial Pain. 2nd ed. Chicago: Quintessence Publishing Co; 1993. pp. 39-60

[43] Stegenga B, De Bont LG, Boering G. Tissue responses to degenerative change in the temporomendibular joint: A review. Journal of Oral and Maxillofacial Surgery. 1991;**49**(10):1079-1088

[44] Milam SB. TMJ osteoarthritis. In: Laskin DM, Greene CS, Hylander WL, editors. Temporomandibular Disorders: An Evidence-Based Approach to Diagnosis and Treatment. Chicago: Quintessence Publishing Co; 2006. pp. 105-123 (ch. 7)

[45] Stegenga B, De Bont LG, Van der Kuijl B, Boering G. Classification of temporomandibular osteoarthrosis and internal derengements. Part I: Diagnostic significance of clinical and radiographic symptoms and signs. Cranio. 1992;**10**(2):96-106

[46] Kalladka M, Quek S, Heir G, Eliav E, Mupparapu M, Viswanath A. Temporomandibular joint osteoarthritis: Diagnosis and long-term conservative management: A topic review. Journal of Indian Prosthodontic Society. 2014;**14**(1):6-15. DOI: 10.1007/s13191-013-0321-3

[47] Israel HA. Internal derangement of the temporomandibular joint: New perspectives on an old problem. Oral and Maxillofacial Surgery Clinics of North America. 2016;**28**(3):313-333. DOI: 10.1016/j.coms.2016.03.009

[48] Felstead AM, Revington PJ. Surgical management of temporomandibular joint ankylosis in ankylosing spondylitis. International Journal of Rheumatology. 2011;**2011**:854167. DOI: 10.1155/2011/854167

[49] Yan YB1, Liang SX, Shen J, Zhang JC, Zhang Y. Current concepts in the pathogenesis of traumatic temporomandibular joint ankylosis. Head & Face Medicine. 2014;**10**:35. DOI: 10.1186/1746-160X-10-35

[50] Song JY, Kim SG, Choi HM, Kim HJ. Severe bony ankylosis of the temporomandibular joint on one side and contralateral adhesion: A case report. Imaging Science in Dentistry. 2015;**45**(2):103-108. DOI: 10.5624/isd.2015.45.2.103

Chapter 8

Oral Parafunction - Aetiology, Implications and Relation to Orthodontic Treatment

Luciene Menrique Corradi and Luiz Eduardo Toledo Avelar

Abstract

Oral parafunction can be defined as an extra-functional action of certain components of the stomatognathic system. The automation of this kind of occurrence that persists in the form of a reflex arc is a denominated habit. The oral parafunctional habits are described as the action of clenching or grinding teeth (bruxism), among others. This work approached bruxism due to its clinical importance. To evaluate the predisposing factors to the development of oral parafunction, the orthodontist should have updated knowledge of the whole process of the phenomenon of bruxism. The purposes of this chapter were about the comprehension of the neurophysiology of bruxism and also about the capacity of structural adaptation of the components of the stomatognathic system, the analysis of its aetiological factors, as well as its implications on the structures of the masticatory system, and the verification of the relation between bruxism and the orthodontic treatment. In conclusion, the nature of that oral habit is multifactorial, which implies extrafunctional demand of neurophysiological mechanisms, whose effects are installed from the rupture of the structural limit of the adaptive capacity of the stomatognathic system, peculiar to each individual. The performance of orthodontic treatment is not related to the development of bruxism.

Keywords: bruxism, parafunction, neurophysiology, orthodontic treatment, stomatognathic system

1. Introduction

Parafunction is any disorder in the action of a particular organ or organ system, often characterised by an overactivity of the physiological action associated with a normal function.

In a dental approach, oral parafunction can be defined as an extra-functional action of certain components of the stomatognathic system. In order to understand it, a more complex scope is necessary, reaching the physiological and neurophysiological action of the entire tract of the stomatognathic system involved, as well as the implications of any disturbances within the normal function, always taking into consideration the aspects of the structural and functional adaptations to which the human organism is subject, within certain limits.

The automation of this type of occurrence that persists in the form of a reflex arc is called a habit. Ferreira [1] defined habit as a lasting disposition acquired by frequent repetition of an act, use and custom.

Oral parafunctional habits are described as grinding or clenching teeth (bruxism), nail biting, finger sucking, chewing objects, abnormal craniocervical-facial posture, among others.

In an orthodontic approach, bruxism should be considered due to the clinical importance of its deleterious effects on the dento-orofacial architecture and the awareness of its increasing prevalence observed in individuals seeking orthodontic treatment.

Its aetiology is quite diverse [2], but it is closely related to the central nervous system (CNS) stimulus and its neurotransmissive mechanisms, as well as psychological-emotional aspects.

The parafunctional action is due to the frequent repetition of a specific function over a prolonged period, which may lead to anatomical alterations [2]. Its implications are several and depend directly on the organic reaction, which is individual and particular.

A clinical significance of the investigation of bruxism lies in its considerable role in the aetiology of pain and temporomandibular dysfunction (TMD) [3–5]. In addition, the increasing prevalence of this parafunctional habit in the population and the deleterious effect it causes to the stomatognathic system represent a strong justification for the current approach [6].

2. Aetiology of parafunction

There is controversy regarding the nature of the aetiology of oral parafunction, that is, whether it is multifactorial or of single origin [6, 7].

However, at present, there is a tendency to agree with a strong psychic-emotional participation and, more recently, for the contribution of the use of certain types of drugs in the aetiopathogenesis of bruxism.

It is understood that psychic-emotional situations such as depression and anxiety modify the perception and the tolerance of the individual in face of physical symptoms and situations triggering stress [8]. Considering the constant state of alert imposed by the mere participation in the current society [9], the professional needs to be aware of the degree of involvement of the aetiology, consequences and implications of the mechanism of oral parafunction in the human organism and, above all, in the individual who will undergo orthodontic treatment.

Regarding the prevalence of bruxism, it is believed that when it occurs in the absence of signs and symptoms resulting from this habit that can occur in an episodic and transient way, it is high. As the effects that are characterised by the collapse of the component structures of the stomatognathic system lead to the search for treatment, the prevalence in a population group does not appear significant [3]. In short, as long as bruxism is performed on a level of subconsciously controlled reflex, this habit is not perceived by the individual, except when it begins to draw attention through its signs and symptoms.

3. Neurophysiological aspects of oral parafunction

All the functions exerted by the masticatory complex depend basically on the mechanism of muscular contraction that is nothing more than a response to a stimulus.

In order to study the neurophysiology of the process involved in parafunction, it is necessary to understand the integration between the main functional and anatomical components of the stomatognathic system and the CNS.

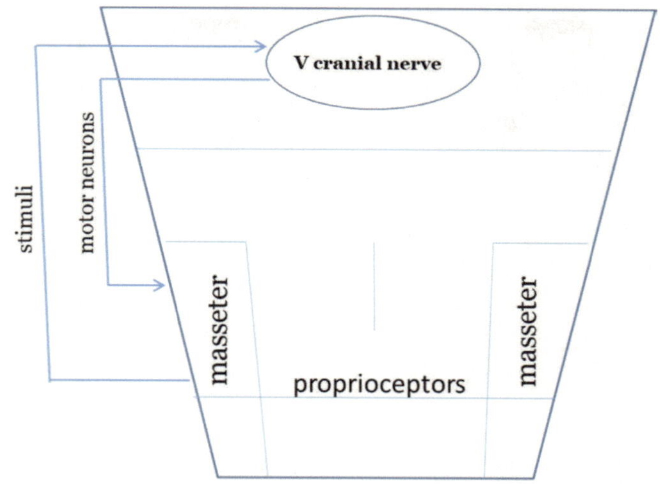

Figure 1.
Reflex action.

The grinding and clenching of teeth are mainly conditioned by the mechanism of muscle contraction. The extra-functional muscular demand caused by bruxism emits stimuli through neuromuscular spindles contained in the intimacy of the muscle fibres that travel through the afferent pathways to the mesencephalic nucleus of the V cranial nerve (trigeminal). From this mesencephalic nucleus, through specific secondary neurons, messages are sent to the trigeminal motor nucleus, located just below, which will send messages via motor neurons to the muscle from which the stimulus started, producing the contraction of its fibres (**Figure 1**) [2].

Although the information is sent to the CNS, the response is independent of the will and normally occurs without the influence of higher centres. This process is known as reflex action [10].

This reflex action occurs through the mechanism called proprioception, which is the term applied to the ability to perceive sensations originating in one's own body. It is a phenomenon linked to cognitive systems of the brain, including memory. The receptors responsible for this function are proprioceptors, which provide information about the position and movement of the mandible and associated oral structures [10].

The parafunctional behaviour is closely related to certain types of stimuli originating in the CNS. These stimuli provoke several organic reactions; among them, the increase of neuromuscular motor excitations, which, in the condition of constant and uninterrupted hyperactivity, is classified as parafunction [11].

4. Organic structural adaptive capacity

All structures of the stomatognathic system, after growth has ceased, are always in the process of transformation and adaptation in conformity with their physiological functional demand, thus conferring a dynamic quality to these structures.

Among the structures of the stomatognathic system is the temporomandibular joint (TMJ). It is subject to functional adaptive changes due to discrepancies that exist between the positions of maximum dental intercuspation and centric relation of the mandible head. These constant TMJ accommodation processes testify to the remarkable adaptability of this joint to adapt to the conflict of these discrepancies, giving the TMJ the characteristic of performing its function in a condition of continuous displacement. No other junction of the human organism has this characteristic [12].

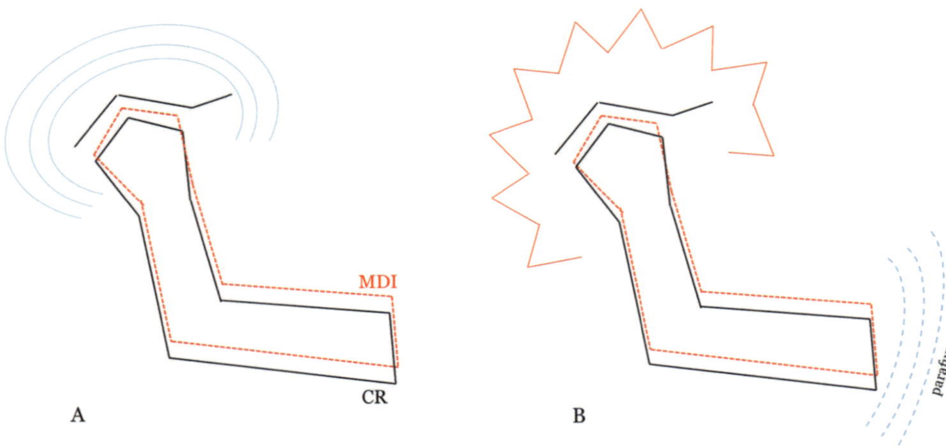

Figure 2.
TMJ accommodation process (A); after the limit of its adaptive capacity has expired, collapses can lead to unpleasant signs and symptoms (B).

Thus, it is understood that the organism, even in the presence of non-physiological situations, exhibits a degree of tolerance in which it has a limiting structural adaptive capacity. That is, after the limit of its adaptive capacity has expired, collapses or even changes in the involved structures can lead to unpleasant signs and symptoms. This is what happens in the mechanism of parafunction (**Figure 2**).

Studies have shown that the bite force performed in episodes of nocturnal bruxism showed an amplitude that exceeded the force that occurred voluntarily during wakefulness and could reach a frequency of four times more [11, 13]. The nocturnal dental contacts during the parafunctional activity can reach a frequency between 15 and 45 minutes of contact between the teeth of the bruxism patients, obtaining, then, an average of 11.4 minutes in these individuals whereas in people without the habit, the average was 3.1 minutes. Thus, it is inferred that the horizontal forces performed in parafunction may have potential to promote adaptations that, associated with other predisposing factors present, determine lesions, since they have a potential much greater than the forces exerted in the physiological function [14].

What modulates the muscular forces and the duration of dental contacts in both the physiological masticatory function and the parafunction is the mechanism of neurological proprioception present in the masticatory system.

There is no functional and anatomical structure in the CNS identifiable as a specific generator of involuntary oromandibular movements [15]. What can be concluded, from the knowledge of the phenomenon of organic adaptability, is that parafunction is a disease that is perceived upon the installation of signs or symptoms related to rupture of the structural limit of the adaptive capacity of the stomatognathic system, particular of each individual.

5. Classification of the oral parafunction

Bruxism can be classified according to severity of symptoms, aetiopathogenesis and clinical manifestations.

The severity of the symptoms depends on the deleterious occurrences on the masticatory system, which present a degree of variability among individuals [6]. This individual variability is conditioned by the organic response, adaptability and predisposition factors represented by the presence of certain deficiencies of the components of the stomatognathic system.

1. Primary
Peripheral: occlusal factors (Ex.: Malocclusion); central: CNS aminergic imbalance (Ex.: Use of SSRIs)
2. Secondary Associated with drugs or other substances (Ex.: Parkinson's disease treatment); associated with sleep disorders (Ex.: Obstructive sleep apnea), neurological disorders (Ex: Akathisia disorder), psychiatric disorders and other diseases
Adapted from Aloé [15].

Table 1.
Classification of bruxism according to its aetiopathogeny.

From another point of view, bruxism can be distinguished according to its aetiopathogenesis, which will lead it basically to two categories: primary and secondary. The primary is the aetiology of bruxism conditioned to peripheral factors due to malocclusion and central factors resulting from neurotransmission disorders [16]. In the secondary category, parafunctional habits associated with clinical, neurological or psychiatric disorders are included, as well as those related to iatrogenic factors, such as in the use or withdrawal of substances or medications, and those resulting from sleep disorders [15] (**Table 1**).

The clinical manifestations represent the signs that denounce the presence of bruxism or its existence for some period, such as the facets of wear and morphology of the dental arches, among others. It is thus perceived that its classification covers the entire process involved in its mechanism, from aetiology to the expression of signs and symptoms.

6. Aetiological considerations of oral parafunction

Bruxism can be considered as a behavioural disorder when considering the prevalence of emotional aetiology. However, when aetiological factors related to organic alterations, such as those occurring in sleep disorders, are considered, it consists of a derangement of the central nervous system [3].

In an analysis of the contribution of peripheral and central factors in the aetiology of bruxism, Lobbezoo and Naeije [17] concluded that there is strong evidence that the role of occlusal features and other morphological factors is small or even null. There is also evidence that disturbances in the central dopaminergic system are implicated in the aetiology of bruxism. In addition, the role of other aetiological factors such as smoking, alcohol, disease, trauma, heredity, stress and other psychological factors is probably lesser than assumed so far. In short, it can be said that bruxism has central and not peripheral mediation [17].

The theory of the combination of peripheral (occlusal) and emotional factors in the aetiology of bruxism is advocated by several authors [6, 14, 17]. Moreover, some drugs such as amphetamines, alcohol, and also sleep disorders, CNS disorders and hereditary factors may be related to the onset of bruxism [6].

Based on these considerations, it is inferred that the multifactorial nature of the aetiology of bruxism can be enumerated in a way to clarify, briefly, each of the main causes of this parafunctional habit increasingly investigated by several research fronts, according to their interests and lines of conduct.

6.1 Emotional factor

Several psychological conditions, such as stress, anxiety or aggressiveness, have been associated with the presence of oral parafunctional habits, which are also recognised as stereotyped movements of the masticatory muscles [18]. An emotional aetiological component, such as psychological stress, may play an important role [19–21], but not all those who grind teeth present emotional problems [21].

The relationship between degrees of dysfunctions of the masticatory system, presence of parafunctional habit and anxiety can be analysed by means of trait-state anxiety scales. Anxiety trait refers to personality trait; anxiety state is defined as a transient emotional state. Thus, there is a positive correlation between the degree of myofascial pain dysfunction (MPD) and the presence of bruxism with the level of anxiety in both scales of trait and state, that is, both an anxious personality and a transient state of anxiety may be directly proportional to the bruxism event and degrees of MPD [22].

Stress is a reaction of the organism to situations of danger that, at first, does not produce deleterious implications. What causes the installation of serious organic complications is uninterrupted stress [11].

In a stress condition, stimuli are routed to the hypothalamus, which in turn activates the pituitary gland, which will sensitise the adrenal gland. The observed reactions can be described as increased blood pressure, gastric problems, insomnia, hair loss and heavy and involuntary isometric contractions of the masticatory muscles. Even though the masticatory muscles are classified as voluntary, their stress contractions may become involuntary through CNS-induced stimuli [11]. Another modification is the creation of additional muscle activity without altering the performance of tasks. These additional activities are considered to be nervous habits, such as bruxism [10].

It is interesting to note that the hypothalamus, in addition to producing the hormone corticotropin to induce the pituitary gland, also activates the cognitive systems of the brain, including memory, to evaluate the stimulus. If the situation that initiated the stimulus poses no danger, the hypothalamus suspends the whole process (**Figure 3**). For this interpretation, it is worth remembering that the body reacts to stress by increasing its metabolism in order to adapt to the new demands. This leads to the decrease in the organic adaptation threshold. This structural tolerance, which is the point at which collapse begins, is an individual characteristic and directly dependent on personality factors. Thus, what differentiates the stressful manifestations in individuals, in general, are these personality factors as radical positions in relation to the facts, competitiveness and the need to dominate situations [11].

For this reason, the individual evaluation becomes essential in the approach of the emotional effects on the parafunction. However, emotional conditions are difficult to become operational in a research because there are many individual

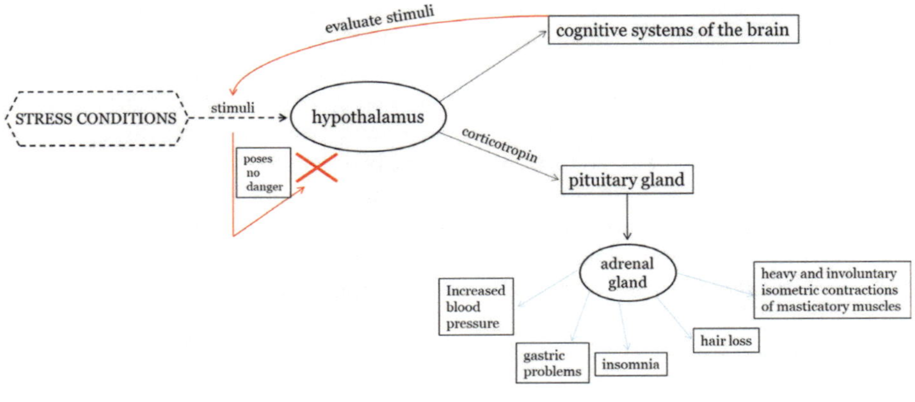

Figure 3.
Stress conditions.

differences in the way the personality and the presence of bruxism are investigated [17]. Thus, it is believed that the participation of emotional factors in the aetiology of this habit may be less than what was previously attributed.

In a study about the relationship between stress level and bruxism using tricyclic antidepressants (amitriptyline) to control pain and stress, there were positive results, that is, the level of stress associated with bruxism was reduced in low doses of this medication [23]. Thus, as previously mentioned, emotional stress has a more significant influence on bruxism than the occlusal factor [7].

Another expression of oral parafunction characterised by grinding or clenching of teeth in an altered emotional condition may attenuate the effects of stress or anxiety on the organism, since in this condition, there are central neurotransmissive changes that can be considered as a strategy to support or even deal with stress and thus minimise its effects on the body [18].

The lack of awareness of the complications that can arise from stressful situations, the lack of perception of the slow and gradual installation of the organic implications of constant stress and the alienation before the management of these situations for a better coexistence converge to the inevitable condition of veritable collapse of important organic structures, such as the stomatognathic system, which can sometimes become irreversible.

6.2 Factors associated with medications and neural pathways

There is evidence that neurochemical factors may be related to the aetiology of bruxism [6]. The acute exposure to stress determines the production of various neurotransmitters such as noradrenaline, dopamine and serotonin [18]. Thus, the involvement of central dopamine in the aetiopathogenesis of parafunctional movements [18] confers the participation of dopaminergic and serotonergic neurotransmission in the genesis and modulation of bruxism [16].

The corpus striatum has the highest concentration of dopamine and is considered the most relevant brain region in the mediation of oral stereotyped movements. Studies in rodents have shown that administration of high doses of dopaminergic agonists (apomorphine) induced oral stereotyped movements such as those occurring in bruxism [18].

Bruxism is primarily a CNS phenomenon, common to all people. In this way, the intensity of the central process responsible for bruxism could be a persistent feature of a person who presents it in childhood and continues to present it in adulthood [24].

Most brain functions are the result of converged actions of various neurotransmitters. The neurotransmitter responsible for inhibiting spontaneous movements of the masticatory muscles and maintaining its tonus is dopamine [16].

Serotonin-concentrating drugs such as selective serotonin reuptake inhibitors (SSRIs) also alter the level of dopamine in the mesocortical tract and frontal cortex [15–17, 25, 26]. This effect can be explained by the effect of these drugs on the dopaminergic system [16, 17]. It is believed that serotonin exerts modulatory influence on dopamine, which is the main neurotransmitter in muscle activity [17].

There are two hypotheses compatible with these changes: hyperdopaminergic and hypodopaminergic. The first may be related to the chronic use of antidopaminergic drugs, such as in the treatment of Parkinson's disease, which causes hypersensitivity of the dopaminergic receptors and may lead to teeth grinding. The second is implicit in the mechanism that occurs with the use of SSRIs: this drug induces the increase of serotonergic transmission that will cause a dopaminergic reduction due to the heteroreceptive serotonin binding on the dopamine receptors of the dopaminergic neurons. In this fashion, there will be a decrease in dopamine binding to its receptors leading to motor disinhibition by the prefrontal cortex and resulting in bruxism. Thus, disordered movements frequently result from elevation of serotonin levels by SSRIs, reducing dopaminergic activity in both the mesocortical and nigrostriatal tracts.

Nevertheless, recent studies indicate that evidence on the manifestation and establishment of drug influences, such as that of the dopamine agonist (pramipexole), on the parafunctional activities of bruxism is inconsistent [27, 28].

There are reports of bruxism induced by other antidepressant medications (venlafaxine, citalopram and SSRIs) that can be controlled with buspirone and gabapentin [15, 16, 29–32]. That is, the use of buspirone can eliminate the bruxism induced by these medicaments due to the restoration of the motor modulation.

Bruxism can be an acute reaction of induction by drugs that increase the level of synaptic serotonin and represent mainly a variation of akathisia. Thus, the diagnosis of bruxism induced by antidepressants may be controversial because of its vague symptoms such as bitemporal headaches, masseter spasm or mandibular pain in addition to classic teeth grinding findings. Therefore, because of its masked presence, bruxism may be much more common than reported [30].

6.3 Occlusal factors

There is controversy regarding the relationship between malocclusion and muscle hyperactivity present in parafunction [11].

What makes it difficult to establish the cause and effect of relationship between these factors is the knowledge of the phenomenon of organic, structural and functional adaptability [11]. As a result of this phenomenon, the divergence of the responses in the individuals is defined as a function of the degree of possible alterations provoked by the muscular hyperactivities for non-functional purposes.

Some authors [33–37] considered that local mechanical factors, especially dental malocclusion, would play a major role in the aetiology of bruxism.

A statistical study performed by Olkinuora [38] found no correlation between the incidence of malocclusion and bruxism.

An analysis of the literature revealed that most of the controversies regarding the role of occlusion in the aetiology of parafunction were derived from inconsistently oriented studies, thus not leading to scientifically defined results. This is due to the difficulty of some researchers to clinically define and stabilise a TMJ position in which the condyles could operate in harmony with the occlusal surfaces of the teeth, preventing a logical and scientific analysis [2].

Stimuli caused by occlusal alterations can generate motor reflex responses by altering the mandibular position and affecting muscle tone [11]. What is understood is that, depending on occlusal interference, its type and location in the occlusal anatomy of the tooth, there may be displacement of the mandible in its closing or eccentric movements, producing unbalanced muscle forces. These mandibular slides, in addition to moving the condyles out of their positions of musculoskeletal stability, may require muscle hyperactivity, altering their tonicity. This may lead to dysfunctions in the stomatognathic system characterised by MPD and orofacial pain involving the whole musculature of the masticatory apparatus [33, 39].

The excess of fatigue and subsequent pain resulting from the sustained contraction of the muscles in the parafunctional activity decreases the threshold of excitability of the neurons of the reflex centre initiating the feedback mechanism. This vicious cycle of the perpetuating increase in muscle tension related to dysfunctional disorders of the teeth, periodontium, TMJ, and masticatory muscles is the basis of bruxism [33].

Based on this reasoning, one could theorise the intrinsic participation of the occlusal factor as a trigger for the parafunctional mechanism. However, it is essential to infer that there will be imbalance of the involved structures if the limit of the organic structural tolerance is broken upon the participation of other supporting aetiological factors, among them the emotional one.

Historically, discrepancies between centric relation and maximum habitual intercuspation and poor tooth positioning were labelled as the most common causes and perpetuating factors of bruxism [17].

Yet, some authors have confirmed the opinion that no occlusal factor alone represents greater importance in the development of TMD and bruxism [40]. Others [6, 33, 36], in contrast, considered the interaction of occlusal and emotional factors as a cause of bruxism.

However, it is believed that there is no scientific evidence that malocclusion or interceptive contact between opposing teeth can initiate or maintain bruxism [3, 14, 32, 41, 42].

In the past, authors such as Ramfjord [33] believed that bruxism should be an instrument with which the individual attempted to eliminate occlusal interference that would cause reflex excitation of the masticatory muscles through stimulation of periodontal mechanoreceptors. However, it is now known that the stimulation of the mechanoreceptors of interceptive dental contacts has a more reduction than increase effect in muscle activity [34, 4–43].

Recently, some studies have demonstrated that the elimination of interferences in occlusion had no influence on parafunctional activity [17, 43–45].

Moreover, not every bruxism patient necessarily presents occlusal interference and those who present it do not always develop the parafunctional habit [17, 35].

The literature points to several controversial theories and opinions regarding the true role of occlusion in the aetiology of bruxism. However, at present, the association between occlusal disharmony and the triggering of bruxism has been debated and challenged, as well as a specific relation between principles of ideal occlusion and absence of bruxism.

What should be considered relevant in relation to the occlusal arrangement during the bruxism mechanism is the distribution of the forces resulting from this activity for non-functional purposes on the teeth and support structures. In a situation of occlusal disharmony, these forces can generate deleterious effects on important components of the masticatory system.

6.4 Other aetiological factors

Other sources in the aetiopathogenesis of oral parafunction are also considered to be factors that trigger bruxism, but no less important in a therapeutic approach [43, 46] such as the aforementioned emotional factors, those associated with medications and neural pathways and occlusal. These are: sleep disorders, genetic factors, use of stimulant and alcoholic beverages and smoking.

6.4.1 Sleep disorders

With regard to sleep disorders, it is understood that during the sleepy state, the use of the masticatory muscles in non-functional activities during the rhythmic attrition of the teeth is characterised as a parafunctional behaviour, that is, it has no functional purpose [3], and thus is believed to be more related to changes in emotional stress levels and sleep stages when neuromuscular protection mechanisms appear to be absent resulting in less influence on muscle activity for non-functional purposes [10, 35, 41, 47].

Night bruxism is common in the general population and represents the third most frequent sleep disorder [21].

As a result of this high prevalence of parafunctional sleep habit, sleep physiology has been studied extensively in order to search for possible causes of this disorder.

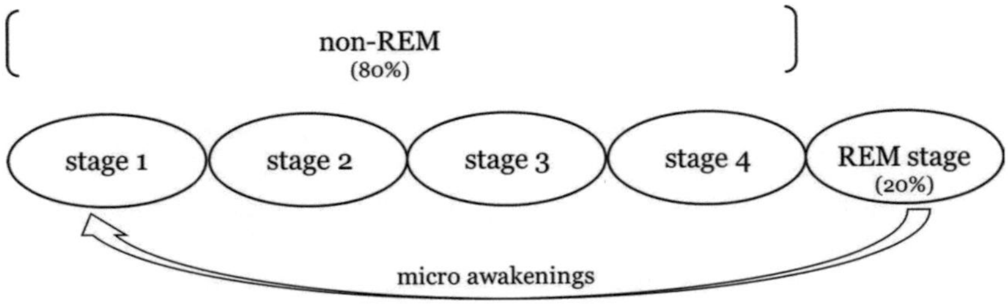

Figure 4.
Adult's sleep period.

The sleep process can be described basically as two types of mental activity: a mild one, which is divided into stages 1 and 2, and a deep one, which is divided into stages 3 and 4. The sequence of these two types of mental activity is called the non-REM phase and represents 80% of an adult's sleep period. The other 20% corresponds to the phase called REM, which is characterised mainly by rapid eye movements. In this way, the sleep cycle is initiated by stages 1 and 2 (superficial), passing to stage 3 (deep) and to stage 4 (even deeper), when it reaches the REM stage. From this REM period, there is a return to the more superficial stage when the so-called micro-awakenings occur. And so the cycle restarts (**Figure 4**) [10].

There is an understanding that nighttime bruxism occurs normally in the non-REM phase, especially in stage 2 and during changes in sleep stages. Nonetheless, there is also another consensus that bruxism may occur during REM sleep and, in this case, is more frequently associated with facial and dental pain [21, 48].

Following this same line of reasoning, there is the theory that parafunctional habit can start at any stage of sleep, but never in its REM stage [36, 49].

Patients with obstructive sleep apnoea, snorers, who present moderate daytime sleepiness, alcoholics, caffeine users, smokers, and those with a highly stressful and anxious life are considered to be at high risk for nighttime bruxism [21].

However, clinical findings showed that there were no significant differences in sleep microstructure in patients with parafunctional habits when compared with individuals considered normal [50].

There are divergences in the literature about which stage of sleep bruxism occurs, such as the observation that bruxism is a relatively nonspecific disturbance of the awakening mechanism, that is, from the passage from sleep to wakefulness. Thus, it can occur as an awakening reaction from any stage [36, 37]. In any case, bruxism is considered a parasomnia, that is, it is a sleep disorder with a high degree of impairment of the structures of the masticatory system, in view of the deficiency of mechanoreceptor mechanisms during the sleep period.

In general, some of the main symptoms that affect people who grind or clench their teeth during sleep are pain in their own teeth, face, head and sensation of muscle fatigue in the areas corresponding to the masseter and temporal muscles that occur in the morning, after awakening and relieving after a few hours [51].

6.4.2 Genetic factors

There are reports of a significant connection of a particular genetic contribution to the pathophysiology of bruxism [21, 38], as well as to the statistically high frequency of the same wear pattern, which reinforces the hypothesis that hereditary factors are important in the genesis and pattern of bruxism and seems to influence the central trigger of this habit [38, 52, 53].

However, in order to establish a pattern of inheritance of the mechanism of bruxism, studies are required encompassing several generations and chromosome identification [54].

6.4.3 Stimulant beverages, tobacco and alcohol

Smoking may increase episodes of tooth grinding during sleep [21]. Both tobacco and stimulant beverages are excitatory substances in the CNS. This means that they may contribute to increase the effect of the stress mechanism, since they present diverse neuromuscular, cardiovascular, and respiratory repercussions. Among stimulating beverages, coffee, tea, chocolate, and cola-based soft drinks may be mentioned [11].

Nicotine also stimulates central dopaminergic activity, which may explain the findings that smokers report bruxism almost twice as often as non-smokers [17, 50, 55]. Alcohol can also induce bruxism [17, 56, 57].

The search for an understanding of the aetiopathogenic basis of bruxism results in diverse and controversial opinions of authors who have studied the subject.

However, it is an almost always present opinion that the aetiological principle of bruxism involves at least two triggering agents and is therefore considered an aetiology of a multifactorial nature.

7. Implications of the mechanism of oral parafunction

Generally, the parafunctional activity for an extended period may imply damage to the structures of the stomatognathic system due to excessive forces applied to the components of this system, which often exceeds the structural tolerance limit of certain structures, as already described.

When the result of the combination of occlusal changes and stress is greater than the body's ability to adapt, muscular hyperactivity is increased, generating intense forces that can reach the structures of the masticatory apparatus, causing collapse [11], that is, this tolerance can be described as a critical level of tolerance to the increased forces generated by the muscular hyperactivity of the components of the masticatory system [10].

Okeson [10] elaborated an equation to demonstrate the aetiology and effect of this muscular hyperactivity :

Malocclusion + Emotional Stress > Physiological Tolerance →

Increased muscle hyperactivity > Structural tolerance → Collapse

This statement reinforces the idea that the response to these situations is individual. The type of reaction is directly related to factors such as particular predisposition to periodontal and dental problems, muscle changes and TMJ. Each one will cause symptomatology originating from its respective deficiency and will give rise to implications on the stomatognathic system, which can also be called biomechanically induced dental diseases. The latter affect at least 75% of the adult population. These data confirm that more teeth are lost due to these diseases than to the effects of caries [12, 58, 59].

There are indications that it is rare to find an individual who presents a condylar and dental relationship with complete balance and harmony. Likewise, an in-depth examination of adults reveals that it is equally rare to find one who has no signs of biomechanically induced dental disease that can be proven to result from grinding and clenching teeth [12].

Following this reasoning, the diagnosis of the presence of the parafunctional habit should be made as early as possible, since in most cases the bruxism patients only suspect its existence when they present damages in the structures of the stomatognathic apparatus, often in a very advanced stage such as dental wear, tooth or restoration fractures, dental hypersensitivity, masticatory muscle discomfort or TMJ pain and in muscles involved in mastication [54].

McCoy [60] used the term dental compression syndrome (DCS) to refer to bruxism and other parafunctional habits such as nail biting. The grinding and clenching of the teeth produce fatigue on the teeth and supporting tissues causing damage to the dental and bone structures and soft and articular tissues. Thus, the understanding of the relationship between DCS and TMD should be further investigated since the effects caused by DCS lead to it becoming an important contributing factor in the onset of TMD and injuries on the teeth [45, 60]. However, there is evidence that clenching teeth (centric bruxism) is more damaging to the masticatory system than grinding teeth (eccentric bruxism) [61].

Among the clinical findings that characterise bruxism, there is a greater predominance of myofascial pain affecting mainly the masseter and the anterior temporalis muscle, followed by dental problems and in the periodontium of support, limitation of the mandibular movements and muscular hypertrophies [62].

The recognition by dentists that bruxism rarely occurs alone, that is, it is always associated with other symptoms, becomes an approach of fundamental importance [63].

What will determine the type of deleterious effects (signs and symptoms) on the stomatognathic system due to the prolonged action of parafunction is the structural tolerance of each component of this system. The potential sites of collapse are the muscles, the TMJs, the supporting structures of the teeth and the teeth themselves.

There is a strong consensus that bruxism is a significant contributing factor in the cause of TMD, including masticatory muscle disorders and joint pain [4–6, 10, 54], such as osteoarthritis, capsulitis, synovitis, disc adhesions and joint pain, in addition to muscle pain [6].

Among the neuromuscular effects that fit the TMDs, one may mention muscle hypertonicity, muscular hypertrophy, movement limitation, myositis and spontaneous myalgia, and myofascial pain. The most frequent symptoms are pain affecting the masseter and anterior temporalis muscles [62, 64].

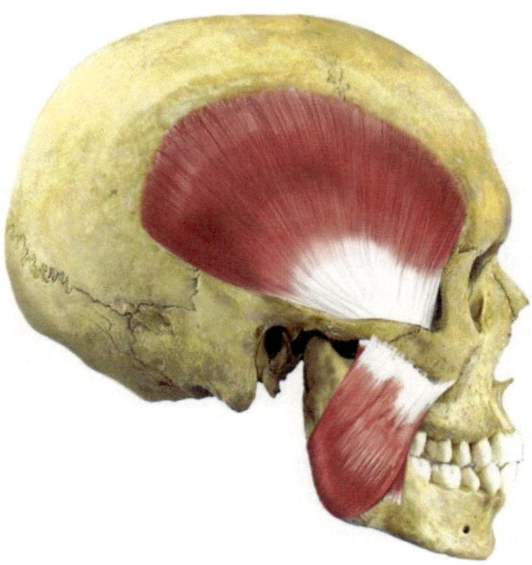

Figure 5.
Main masticatory muscles involved in bruxism: masseter and temporal.

One can also attribute as implications of bruxism the increase in muscle tone and resistance to manipulation of the mandible, in addition to compensatory hypertrophy, muscular fatigue sensation and pain to the palpation of the mastication muscles [36].

7.1 Most frequent symptoms of TMDs

Once the imbalance of the stomatognathic system is established due to oral parafunction, the main symptoms are limitation of physiological activity, noises and pain in TMJ, muscular pain, and limitation and deviation of mandibular movements [65]. However, the mandibular elevating masticatory muscles, especially the masseter and temporal, are the most affected structures in TMDs due to bruxism (**Figure 5**) [65, 66].

TMDs may also be associated with anatomical, physiological and psychological factors, as well as headaches and neck and ear pains [65–67].

8. Changes in morphological craniofacial architecture

Research on the relationship between form (or structure) and function of the components of the masticatory system is of extreme scientific interest because it can elucidate how structures develop beyond their genetic component.

In the case of the extra-functional demand of bruxism, can it exert influence on the craniofacial structures of the individuals who are growing or even those who have passed this stage?

In this context, the craniofacial morphology could perhaps represent one of the signs of some relevance for the clinician to search for. However, the literature shows different opinions, even going to the controversies on this subject.

In 1994, Menapace et al. [68] mentioned that some authors advocated the hypothesis that bruxism directs towards a particular craniofacial morphology and that other researchers, on the contrary, believed that a certain craniofacial morphology may predispose to the parafunctional mechanism. However, when investigating the type of craniofacial and dental morphology between individuals with and without bruxism, these authors did not find significant differences between the two groups.

In a recent study, it was observed that some adult individuals, that is, after the period of facial growth and development, may develop anterior open bite due to episodes of parafunctional oral activity [69].

In another study on the relationship between craniofacial morphology and bruxism, Young et al. [70] found a statistically significant difference in the bizygomatic and cranial widths when they compared bruxism patients with those who did not present the habit. They associated this finding with the theory that the increase in non-functional demand that occurs in bruxism can result in broader or wider skull-and-mouth traits as prescribed by functional matrix theory. Perhaps, the result of these studies indicated a greater functional effect of the masseter and temporal muscles on the skeletal traits of bruxism patients. However, these authors also affirmed that this evidence is based on an indirect rather than a direct premise, since independent variables reported in bruxism were evaluated, such as muscle strength, tooth wear, number and density of muscle fibres and occlusion.

Other data found in research focused on the relationship between tooth wear occurring in bruxism, and the morphology of craniofacial structures was more rectangular maxillary arch in combination with anterior mandibular rotation, diminished anterior facial height and greater bimaxillary interincisal angle [17, 71].

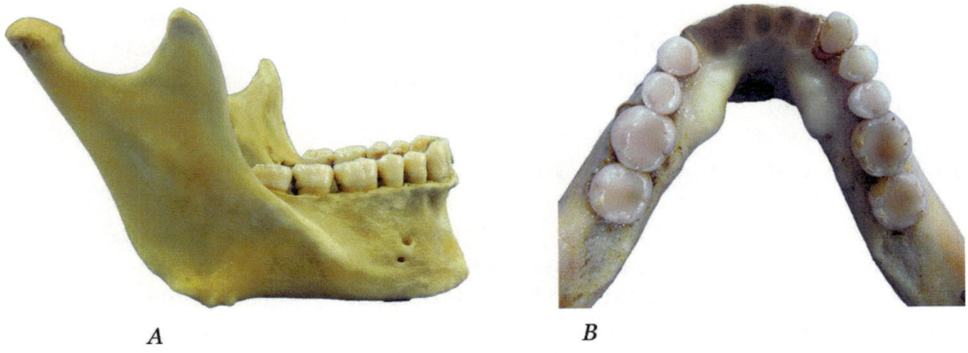

Figure 6.
Prominence of mandibular angle (A); mandibular torus on lingual surface (B).

Other authors [17, 70, 72] believe that parafunctional habit does not imply alteration of facial morphology, since dentoalveolar development should compensate for tooth wear related to bruxism and, therefore, deny a possible effect of reducing facial anterior height in bearers of this habit. Thus, they demonstrated that there is maintenance of the overbite due to the extrusion of anterior teeth so that the contact with its antagonists remains.

Otherwise, alterations of some facial structures can take place, like the prominence of mandibular angle (masseter insertion) and mandibular torus on the lingual surface (**Figure 6**) [73].

From the above, it is observed that there is no consensus on the actual association between craniofacial morphology and the presence of bruxism, and this probable clinical sign consequent to the parafunctional habit should be carefully examined.

9. Therapeutic strategies to control bruxism

Considering the multifactorial aetiological nature of oral parafunction, as well as the different forms of involvement on the dentofacial structures involved, once it is perceived that when the structural limit of the adaptive capacity of the stomatognathic system, which is individual, is reached, the therapeutic approach becomes complex and at the same time palliative. It can be said that bruxism can be controlled by means of different therapeutic procedures on the signs and symptoms resulting from its installation, which is slow and gradual.

The proposed therapeutic strategies can be listed as psychological approach, guidelines on sleep hygiene measures combined with relaxation methods, use of interocclusal devices, prescription of medication for pain control, electrical stimulation, physiotherapy, acupuncture and, more recently, use of botulinum toxin to control the contraction of the main muscles involved in the parafunction, decreasing muscular strength and pain [66, 74–76].

There are currently questions about the influence of the use of invisible orthodontic aligners on the effects of bruxism with regard to parafunctional muscle activity during sleep and, consequently, related symptoms, such as pain. These devices are compared with those used in the traditional therapy of nocturnal bruxism control: hard-resin appliances. The latter provide a decrease in the force of muscle contraction, thus relieving pain symptoms and protecting teeth and structures of the temporomandibular joint. There is no scientific evidence that invisible orthodontic aligners can exert some effect on parafunctional muscle activity during sleep, nor on related symptoms [77].

10. Relation to orthodontic treatment

It is relevant to investigate the real relationship between orthodontic treatment and parafunctional habit, since it is not uncommon for an individual to seek correction of malocclusion in order to solve problems caused by bruxism or even to intercept its own mechanism.

On the other hand, in some cases it may develop the habit of grinding or clenching the teeth during or after orthodontic treatment.

What, then, is the association between orthodontic treatment and bruxism? Is orthodontic treatment responsible for TMD signs and symptoms resulting from parafunction? Can orthodontic therapy be considered as a triggering factor of the parafunctional mechanism? How to evaluate, predict and verify the presence of predisposing factors to parafunction in an individual who will undergo orthodontic treatment?

These issues have been raised, both by individuals who will undergo orthodontic treatment and by professionals themselves, because of a growing prevalence of bruxism currently observed.

To evaluate the factors predisposing to the development of parafunction, the orthodontist must have updated knowledge of the whole process of the phenomenon of bruxism. This encompasses from the neurophysiological criteria of the whole mechanism (CNS control) to the problems related to the aetiology and its implications.

The diversity of factors capable of deflagrating, maintaining or aggravating the mechanism of bruxism and its sequelae requires the orthodontist to know and understand the mechanism of this parafunctional habit in order to have success and clarity in clinical behaviour in relation to individuals who have or who develop it before, during or after orthodontic treatment.

A longitudinal study by Knight et al. [8] for a period of 20 years in individuals receiving orthodontic treatment showed that they presented signs of bruxism characterised by wear in the mixed dentition that remained with the same pattern in the permanent dentition. They inferred that this parafunctional habit may represent a persistent characteristic in the childhood and in the adult phase of the same person, thus not having a direct relation between orthodontic treatment and bruxism.

In another study, Egermark et al. [40] investigated the risk of developing bruxism and TMD in a group of 402 subjects, some of whom received orthodontic treatment while others represented the control group. The results reinforced the opinion that orthodontic treatment did not present a high risk of developing TMD and bruxism in the long term when compared to those who did not undergo orthodontic intervention to correct malocclusion.

In contrast, there are reports that bruxism and some signs and symptoms of TMD have decreased during the active phase of orthodontic treatment [78].

A possible explanation for the association between these two entities is based on the understanding of the neurophysiology of the CNS involved in its processes.

According to Okeson [10], the constant change of the dental positions in the orthodontic conduct results in altered peripheral sensorial stimuli causing a decrease of CNS activity. That is, occlusal contacts generate peripheral (outside the CNS) stimuli, which present an inhibitory effect of muscle activity through the nociceptive reflex mechanism. In a different way, bruxism seems to be conditioned to the CNS, whose stimulus has an excitatory effect on the muscles.

Thus, it can be inferred that the muscular activities related to functional (occlusion) and parafunctional (bruxism) stimuli are different, as they result in controlled and voluntary movements and uncontrolled and involuntary movements, respectively. From this reasoning, it can be deduced that changes in dental contacts have little effect on bruxism, that is, as the teeth move in orthodontic treatment, they produce constant peripheral stimuli that act to inhibit parafunctional activity, which is mediated mainly by the CNS. However, once the orthodontic movements have settled, if the main aetiological factor persists, bruxism may restart [10]. Likewise, the effect of therapy using rigid plaques that are constantly adjusted to control the habit and protect the structures associated with the parafunctional act, such as teeth, neuromuscular structures and TMJ, is understood.

This hypothesis is contradictory in relation to the authors who defended the occlusion and its variations as one of the main triggers of bruxism [33]. On the other hand, it supports the results of studies of other researchers who found a reduction in parafunctional muscle activity after the inclusion of deflective occlusal contacts in a given population sample [79].

At present, there is a concern to investigate the real participation of orthodontic treatment in the development of one of the consequences of bruxism represented by TMD.

Studies have demonstrated that parafunctional habits can act as triggers for TMD, that is, they are conditioned by the contributing factors of these disorders, as revealed by Conti [4] in a cross-sectional evaluation of the relationship between TMD signs and symptoms and orthodontic treatment.

Other authors have claimed that parafunctional habits do not represent consistent factors in the induction of muscle or joint pathologies [80].

In this way, one cannot neglect the fact that the uncertainty caused by the lack of scientific evidence based on subsidies of greater content around the true involvement of orthodontics on the parafunctional mechanism converges to a more prudent conduct in relation to orthodontic procedures in patients with bruxism.

Clinical examination, diagnosis and discernment to know the timing to initiate or continue orthodontic treatment in patients who are included in this context constitute adequate procedures to conduct the orthodontic intervention.

Some professionals postpone the control and treatment of bruxism only after removal of the fixed appliance, even though this may result in excessive tooth wear. Others advocate some type of control for the consequences of bruxism during orthodontic treatment, such as the use of occlusal plaques [81].

In a longitudinal follow-up of a sample composed of 58 TMD patients, of whom 45 were submitted to orthodontic treatment, Imai et al. [82] suggested that TMD-related symptoms did not recur in individuals receiving orthodontic treatment due, probably, to the reestablishment of the functional balance of the masticatory system.

These data are consistent with the idea that a healthy occlusal condition is essential for the entire dynamics of the stomatognathic system. Otherwise, along with other triggering factors, a situation of occlusal disharmony can act as an aggravating factor of the deleterious phenomena originated by bruxism.

From this, studies have shown that the relationship between tooth movement and the aetiological mechanism of parafunctional habits is inconsistent.

Therefore, the researched literature did not provide scientific support for the hypothesis of a direct association between bruxism and orthodontic treatment, which reinforces the need for further research on this subject.

11. Conclusions

This chapter dealt with aspects related to the aetiology of oral parafunction, as well as related neurophysiology, organic structural adaptive capacity, some clinical implications such as the main structures of the stomatognathic system involved consequent to the TMDs, alterations in the craniofacial morphological architecture, some therapeutic conducts and, finally, the association between orthodontic treatment and bruxism.

The aetiology of bruxism is multifactorial. The deleterious events on the cranio-orofacial architecture come from the rupture of the structural limit of the adaptive capacity of the stomatognathic system as a consequence of the oral parafunction, and it is particular of each individual. However, the facial structures that are most affected by bruxism are the mandibular elevating masticatory muscles: masseter and temporal. The therapeutic conducts used to control bruxism should be directed in accordance with the prevalence of each symptomatology, as well as according to the specific aetiology. Finally, orthodontic treatment cannot be considered as an aetiological factor of bruxism, since occlusal interferences are no longer accepted as the main aetiological factor in this occurrence. Following this reasoning, it can be concluded that the performance of orthodontic treatment is not related to the presence of signs and symptoms of temporomandibular disorders (TMD), since the degree of TMD may be associated with the presence of parafunctional habits (such as bruxism and clenching of teeth) and emotional tension.

Thus, knowledge and mastery of signs and symptoms of bruxism, in addition to contributing factors in its aetiology, as well as knowledge about the different therapeutic approaches, become fundamental requirements, within a more current perspective, in the practice of orthodontics.

Author details

Luciene Menrique Corradi* and Luiz Eduardo Toledo Avelar
Anthropologist of Police Department of Minas Gerais State, Instituto Médico Legal, Belo Horizonte, Brazil

*Address all correspondence to: lumcorradi@gmail.com

References

[1] Ferreira ABH. Dicionário Aurélio básico da língua portuguesa. São Paulo: Nova Fronteira; 1994-1995. p. 687

[2] Paiva HJ. Oclusão: Noções e Conceitos Básicos. São Paulo: Santos; 1997

[3] Leles CR, Melo M. Bruxismo e apertamento dental—Uma conduta clínica racional. Revista Odontológica do Brasil-Central. 1995;**5**(15):22-26

[4] Conti ACCF. Avaliação transversal da relação entre sinais e sintomas das disfunções têmporo-mandibulares e o tratamento ortodôntico [Dissertação de Mestrado]. Bauru: Faculdade de Odontologia da USP; 2000

[5] Rodrigues L, Lemos JBD, Tokura M, Luz JGC. Freqüência de hábitos parafuncionais e suas manifestações clínicas em pacientes com disfunções da articulação temporomandibular. Revista de Odontologia da Universidade Cidade de São Paulo. 2001;**13**(2):113-123

[6] Uetanabara R, Mazzetto MO. Bruxism: A current view. Revista de Odontologia da Universidade Cidade de São Paulo. 2000;**12**(2):163-169

[7] Pavarina AC, Bussadori CMC, Alencar FGP Jr. Aspectos dos hábitos parafuncionais de interesse para o clínico geral. Journal Brasileiro de Odontologia Clínica. 1999;**3**(13):86-90

[8] Knight DJ, Leroux BG, Zhu C, Almond J, Ramsay DS. A longitudinal study of tooth wear in orthodontically treated patients. American Journal of Orthodontics and Dentofacial Orthopedics. 1997;**112**(2):194-202. DOI: 10.1016/S0889-5406(97)70246-4

[9] Pinheiro M. Era da Ansiedade. Estado de Minas, Belo Horizonte, Feminino & Masculino; 2002. p. 8

[10] Okeson JP. Fundamentos de Oclusão e Desordens Têmporo-Mandibulares. Trad. de Milton Edson Miranda. 2nd ed. São Paulo: Artes Médicas; 1992

[11] Maciel RN, Gomes SS. Oclusão e ATM: Procedimentos Clínicos. 2nd ed. São Paulo: Santos; 1996

[12] Simon J. Biomechanically-induced dental disease. General Dentistry. 2000;**48**(5):598-605

[13] Nishigawa K, Bando E, Nakano N. Quantitative study of bite force during sleep association bruxism. Journal of Oral Rehabilitation. 2001;**28**(5):485-491. DOI: 10.1046/j.1365-2842.2001.00692.x

[14] Kydd WL, Daly C. Duration of nocturnal tooth contacts during bruxing. The Journal of Prosthetic Dentistry. 1985;**53**(5):717-721. DOI: 10.1016/0022-3913(85)90031-9

[15] Aloé F, Gonçalves LR, Azevedo A, Barbosa RC. Sleep bruxism. Reviews Neuroscience. 2003;**11**(1):4-17

[16] Bostwick JM, Jaffee MS. Buspirone as an antidote to SSRI-induced bruxism in 4 cases. The Journal of Clinical Psychiatry. 1999;**60**(12):857-860

[17] Lobbezoo F, Naeije M. Bruxism is mainly regulated centrally, not peripherally. Journal of Oral Rehabilitation. 2001;**28**(12):1085-1089. DOI: 10.1046/j.1365-2842.2001.00839.x

[18] Gómez FM, Giralt MT, Sainz B, Arrue A, Prieto M, García-Vallejo P. A possible attenuation of stress-induced increases in striatal dopamine metabolism by the expression of non-functional masticatory in the rat. European Journal of Oral Sciences. 1999;**107**(6):461-467. DOI: 10.1046/j.0909-8836.1999.eos107607.x

[19] Arman K, Petruninaitė A, Grigalauskienė R. Stress experience

and effect on self-perceived oral health status among high school students. Stomatologija. 2016;**18**(3):75-79

[20] Alves AC, Alchieri JC, Barbosa GAS. Bruxism. Masticatory implications and anxiety. Acta Odontológica Latinoamericana. 2013;**26**(1):15-22

[21] Ohayon MM, Li KK, Guilleminault C. Risk factors for sleep bruxism in the general population. Chest. 2001;**119**(1):53-61. DOI: 10.1378/chest.119.1.53

[22] Alencar Junior FGP. Fatores psicológicos nas disfunções craniomandibulares: estudo da relação entre graus de disfunção e escalas de ansiedade traço-estado [Dissertação de Mestrado]. Bauru: Faculdade de Odontologia da USP; 1997

[23] Raigrodski AJ, Mohamed SE, Gardiner DM. The effect of amitriptyline on pain intensity and perception of stress in bruxers. Journal of Prosthodontics. 2001;**10**(2):73-77. DOI: 10.1111/j.1532-849X.2001.00073.x

[24] Seligman DA, Pullinger AG, Solber WK. The prevalence of dental attrition and its association with factors of age, gender, occlusion and TMJ symptomatology. Journal of Dental Research. 1988;**67**(10):1323-1333. DOI: 10.1177/00220345880670101601

[25] Baldessarini RJ, Marsh E. Fluoxetine and side effects. Archives of General Psychiatry. 1990;**47**(2):191-192. DOI: 10.1001/archpsyc.1990.01810140091015

[26] Possidente E, Nardi AE, Figueira I, Mendlowicz M, Marques C, Versiani M. SSRI-associated bruxism: Case report of 4 patients. Jornal Brasileiro de Psiquiatria. 1997;**46**(5):285-288

[27] Macedo CR, Macedo EC, Torloni MR, Silva AB, Prado GF. Pharmacotherapy for sleep bruxism. Cochrane Database of Systematic Reviews. 2014;**23**(10):CD005578. DOI: 10.1002/14651858.CD005578.pub2

[28] Cahlin BJ, Hedner J, Dahlström L. A randomised, open-label, crossover study of the dopamine agonist, pramipexole, in patients with sleep bruxism. Journal of Sleep Research. 2017;**26**(1):64-72. DOI: 10.1111/jsr.12440

[29] Ellison JM, Stanziani P. SSRI—Associated nocturnal bruxism in four patients. The Journal of Clinical Psychiatry. 1993;**54**(11):432-434

[30] Jaffee MS, Bostwick JM. Buspirone as an antidote to venlafaxine-induced bruxism. Psychosomatics. 2000;**41**(6): 535-536. DOI: 10.1176/appi.psy.41.6.535

[31] Wise MEJ. Citalopram-induced bruxism. The British Journal of Psychiatry. 2001;**178**:182. DOI: 10.1192/bjp.178.2.182

[32] Brown ES, Hong SC. Antidepressant-induced bruxism successfully treated with gabapentin. Journal of the American Dental Association. 1999;**130**(10):1467-1469. DOI: 10.14219/jada.archive.1999.0057

[33] Ramfjord SP. Bruxism, a clinical and electromyographic study. Journal of the American Dental Association. 1961;**62**:21-44. DOI: 10.14219/jada.archive.1961.0002

[34] Strother EW, Mitchell GE. Bruxism: A review and a case report. The Journal of Dental Medicine. 1954;**9**:189

[35] Wigdorowicz-Makowerowa N, Godzki C, Panek H, Maslanka T, Plonka K, Palacha A. Epidemiological study on prevalence and etiology of functional disturbances of the masticatory system. The Journal of Prosthetic Dentistry. 1979;**41**(1):76. DOI: 10.1016/0022-3913(79)90361-5

[36] Reimão R, Lefèvre AB. Prevalence of nocturnal bruxism in childhood.

Revista do Hospital das Clínicas Universidade de São Paulo Hospital das Clínicas. 1982;**37**(5):228-232

[37] Funato M, Ono Y, Baba K, Kudo Y. Evaluation of the non-functional tooth contact in patients with temporomandibular disorders by using newly developed electronic system. Journal of Oral Rehabilitation. 2014;**41**(3):170-176. DOI: 10.1111/joor.12129

[38] Olkinuora M. Bruxism: A review of the literature on and a discussion of studies of bruxism and its psychogenesis and some new psychological hypotheses. Suomen Hammaslääkäriseuran Toimituksia. 1969;**65**(6):312-324

[39] Rosara JV, Barbosa TS, Dias IOV, Kobayashi FY, Costa YM, Gavião MBD, et al. Effect of interocclusal appliance on bite force, sleep quality, salivary cortisol levels and signs and symptoms of temporomandibular dysfunction in adults with sleep bruxism. Archives of Oral Biology. 2017;**82**:62-70. DOI: 10.1016/j.archoralbio.2017.05.018

[40] Egermark I, Magnusson T, Carlsson GE. A 20-year follow-up of signs and symptoms of temporomandibular disorders and malocclusions in subjects with and without orthodontic treatment in childhood. The Angle Orthodontist. 2003;**73**(2):109-115. DOI: 10.1043/0003-3219(2003)73<109:AYFOSA>2.0.CO;2

[41] Clarke NG. Occlusion and myofascial pain dysfunction: Is there a relatioship? Journal of the American Dental Association. 1982;**104**:443-446. DOI: 10.14219/jada.archive.1982.0233

[42] Vanderas AP, Manetas KJ. Relationship between malocclusion and bruxism in children and adolescents: A review. Pediatric Dentistry. 1995;**17**(1):7-12

[43] Dalewski B, Chrusciel-Nogalska M, Frazczak B. Occlusal splint versus modified nociceptive trigeminal inhibition splint in bruxism therapy: A randomized, controlled trial using surface electromyography. Australian Dental Journal. 2015;**60**(4):445-454. DOI: 10.1111/adj.12259

[44] Kardachi BJR, Bailey JO, Ash MM. A comparision of biofeedback and occlusal adjustment on bruxism. Journal of Periodontology. 1978;**49**:367. DOI: 10.1902/jop.1978.49.7.367

[45] Bailey JO, Rugh JD. Effect of occlusal adjustment on bruxism as monitired by nocturnal EMG recordings. Journal of Dental Research. 1980;**59**:317. DOI: 10.1016/0022-3913(81)90207-9

[46] Kuhn M, Türp JC. Risk factors for bruxism: A review of the literature from 2007 to 2016. Swiss Dental Journal. 2018;**128**(2):118-124

[47] Shinkai RSA, Santos LM, Silva FA, Santos MN. Prevalence of nocturnal bruxismin 2-11-year-old children. Revista de Odontologia da Universidade Cidade de São Paulo. 1998;**12**(1):29-37. DOI: 10.1590/S0103-06631998000100006

[48] Carra MC, Macaluso GM, Rompré PH, Huynh N, Parrino L, Terzano MG, et al. Clonidine has a paradoxical effect on cyclic arousal and sleep bruxism during NREM sleep. Sleep. 2010;**33**(12):1711-1716. DOI: 10.1093/sleep/33.12.1711

[49] Satoh T, Harada Y. Electrophysiological study on tooth-grinding during sleep. Electroencephalography and Clinical Neurophysiology. 1973;**35**(3):267-275. DOI: 10.1016/0013-4694(73)90238-1

[50] Lavigne GJ, Rompré PH, Guitard F, Sessle BJ, Kato T, Montplaisir JY. Lower number of K-complexes and K-alphas in sleep bruxism: A controlled quantitative

study. Clinical Neurophysiology. 2002;**113**(5):686-693. DOI: 10.1016/S1388-2457(02)00037-8

[51] Silva SR. Bruxismo. Revista da Associação Paulista de Cirurgiões Dentistas. 2003;**57**(6):409-417

[52] Abe K, Shimakawa M. Genetic and developmental aspects of sleep talking and teeth-grinding. Acta Paedopsychiatrica. 1966;**33**(11):339-344

[53] Lindqvist B. Bruxism in twins. Acta Odontologica Scandinavica. 1974;**32**(3):177-187. DOI: 10.3109/00016357409002546

[54] Kato T, Thie NMR, Montplaisir JY, Lavigne GJ. Bruxism and orofacial movements during sleep. Dental Clinics of North America. 2001;**45**(4):657-684

[55] Madrid G, Madrid S, Vranesh JG, Hicks RA. Cigarette smoking and bruxism. Perceptual and Motor Skills. 1998;**87**(3 Pt 1):898. DOI: 10.2466/pms.1998.87.3.898

[56] Lavigne GJ, Lobbezzo F, Rompré PH, Nielsen TA, Montplaisir JY. Cigarette smoking as a risk or exacerbating factor for restless legs syndrome and sleep bruxism. Sleep. 1997;**20**(4):290-293. DOI: 10.1093/sleep/20.4.290

[57] Hartman E. Bruxism. In: Kryger MH, Roth T, Dement WC, editors. Principles and Practice of Sleep Medicine. 2nd ed. Philadelphia: W. B. Saunders; 1994. pp. 598-601

[58] Alharby A, Alzayer H, Almahlawi A, Alrashidi Y, Azhar S, Sheikho M, et al. Parafunctional behaviors and its effect on dental bridges. Journal of Clinical Medical Research. 2018;**10**(2):73-76. DOI: 10.14740/jocmr3304w

[59] Kawakami S, Kumazaki Y, Manda Y, Oki K, Minagi S. Specific diurnal EMG activity pattern observed in occlusal collapse patients: Relationship between diurnal bruxism and tooth loss progression. PLoS One. 2014;**9**(7):e101882. DOI: 10.1371/journal.pone.0101882

[60] McCoy G. Dental compression syndrome: A new look at an old disease. The Journal of Oral Implantology. 1999;**25**(1):35-49. DOI: 10.1563/1548-1336(1999)025<0035:DCSANL>2.3.CO;2

[61] Kampe T, Tagdae T, Bader G, Edman G, Karlsson S. Reported symptoms and clinical findings in a group of subjects with longstanding bruxing behaviour. Journal of Oral Rehabilitation. 1997;**24**(8):581-587. DOI: 10.1111/j.1365-2842.1997.tb00377.x

[62] Fernandes RSM, Mazzetto MO. Achados clínicos que caracterizam o bruxismo em pacientes com queixas de desordens crânio-mandibulares. In: Anais. Vol. 21. Ribeirão Preto: FORP-USP; 1999. p. 52

[63] Muzyka BC. Sleep bruxism—New findings. Practical Procedures & Aesthetic Dentistry. 2001;**13**(3):190

[64] Arita CA, Carvalho PCL, Silva MAMR, Bataglion C, Chaguri NA, Nunes LJ. Alterações provocadas pelo bruxismo. RGO. 1990;**38**(4):257-261

[65] Garip H, Tufekcioglu S, Kaya E. Changes in the temporomandibular joint disc and temporal and masseter muscles secondary to bruxism in Turkish patients. Saudi Medical Journal. 2018;**39**(1):81-85. DOI: 10.15537/smj.2018.1.20873

[66] Asutay F, Atalay Y, Asutay H, Acar AH. The evaluation of the clinical effects of botulinum toxin on nocturnal bruxism. Pain Research & Management. 2017;**2017**:6264146. DOI: 10.1155/2017/6264146

[67] Lund JP et al. Dor Orofacial: Da Ciência Básica à Conduta Clínica. São Paulo: Quintessence; 2010. p. 300

[68] Menapace SE, Rinchuse DJ, Zullo T, Pierce CJ, Shnorhokian H. The

dentofacial morphology of bruxers versus non-bruxers. The Angle Orthodontist. 1994;**64**(1):43-52. DOI: 10.1043/0003-3219(1994)064<0043:TDMOBV>2.0.CO;2

[69] Broberg K, Lindskog-Stokland B, Mejersjö C. Anterior bite opening in adulthood. The Open Dentistry Journal. 2017;**11**:628-635. DOI: 10.2174/1874210601711010628

[70] Young DV, Rinchuse DJ, Pierce CJ, Zullo T. The craniofacial morphology of bruxers versus nonbruxers. The Angle Orthodontist. 1999;**69**(1):14-18. DOI: 10.1043/0003-3219(1999)069<0014:TCMOBV>2.3.CO;2

[71] Waltimo A, Nyström M, Könönen M. Bite force and dentofacial morphology in men with severe dental attrition. Scandinavian Journal of Dental Research. 1994;**102**(2):92. DOI: 10.1111/j.1600-0722.1994.tb01161.x

[72] Crothers A, Sandham A. Vertical height differences in subjects with severe dental wear. European Journal of Orthodontics. 1993;**15**(6):519-525. DOI: 10.1093/ejo/15.6.519

[73] Clifford T, Lamey PJ, Fartash L. Mandibular tori, migraine and temporomandibular disorders. British Dental Journal. 1996;**180**(10):382-384. DOI: 10.1038/sj.bdj.4809094

[74] Jadhao VA, Lokhande N, Habbu SG, Sewane S, Dongare S, Goyal N. Efficacy of botulinum toxin in treating mofascial pain and occlusal force characteristics of masticatory muscles in bruxism. Indian Journal of Dental Research;**201728**(5):493-497. DOI: 10.4103/ijdr.IJDR_125_17

[75] Salgueiro MDCC, Bortoletto CC, Horliana ACR, Mota ACC, Motta LJ, Motta PB, et al. Evaluation of muscle activity, bite force and salivary cortisol in children with bruxism before and after low level laser applied to acupoints: Study protocol for a randomised controlled trial. BMC Complementary and Alternative Medicine. 2017;**17**(1):391. DOI: 10.1186/s12906-017-1905-y

[76] Kesikburun S, Alaca R, Aras B, Tuğcu I, Tan AK. Botulinum toxin injection for bruxism associated with brain injury: Case report. Journal of Rehabilitation Research and Development. 2014;**51**(4):661-664. DOI: 10.1682/JRRD.2013.10.0218

[77] Manfredini D, Lombardo L, Vigiani L, Arreghini A, Siciliani G. Effects of invisible orthodontic retainers on masticatory muscles activity during sleep: A controlled trial. Progress in Orthodontics. 2018;**19**(1):24. DOI: 10.1186/s40510-018-0228-y

[78] Egermark I, Rönnerman A. Temporomandibular disorders in the active phase of orthodontic treatment. Journal of Oral Rehabilitation. 1995;**22**(8):613-618. DOI: 10.1111/j.1365-2842.1995.tb01058.x

[79] Rugh JD, Barghi N, Drago CJ. Experimental occlusal discrepancies and nocturnal bruxism. The Journal of Prosthetic Dentistry. 1984;**51**(4):548-553. DOI: 10.1016/0022-3913(84)90312-3

[80] Barne A, Sbordone L, Ramaglia L. Craniomandibular disorders and orthodontic treatment need in children. Journal of Oral Rehabilitation. 1997;**24**(1):2-7. DOI: 10.1111/j.1365-2842.1997.tb00252.x

[81] Sullivan TC. A new occlusal splint for treating bruxism and TMD during orthodontic therapy. Journal of Clinical Orthodontics. 2001;**35**(3):142-144

[82] Imai T, Okamoto T, Kaneko T, Umeda K, Yamamoto T, Nakamura S. Long-term follow-up of clinical symptoms in TMD patients who underwent occlusal reconstruction by orthodontic treatment. European Journal of Orthodontics. 2000;**22**(1):61-67

Section 3

Psychosocial Effect of Maxillofacial Deformities

Chapter 9

The Effects of Maxillomandibular Advancement and Genioglossus Advancement on Sleep Quality

Takako Sato, Ryota Nakamura, Akio Himejima, Akemi Kusano, Serim Kang, Saori Ohtani, Kentarou Yamada, Kanako Yamagata, Hiroaki Azaki, Junya Aoki, Keiichi Yanagawa, Keiji Shinozuka, Takeya Yamada and Morio Tonogi

Abstract

Maxillomandibular advancement (MMA) using a standardized surgical procedure consisting of a LeFort I osteotomy and bilateral sagittal split ramus osteotomy and genioglossus advancement (GA) using a genioplasty improve airway volume, oxygen desaturation, and the AHI in patients with OSA. However, there are few reports on changes in sleep quality following MMA and GA. We assessed the effects of MMA and GA on sleep quality by comparing oxygen desaturation, AHI, and sleep architecture before and after surgery. Methods: Eight patients underwent polysomnography (PSG) and CT scan before and after surgery. Conclusions: Our study finds that %TST and %REM were both increased, while %S1 and NA both decreased. Based on these results, it appears that both the quality and quantity of sleep were improved. MMA and GA improve sleep respiratory disturbance and can also improve sleep quality.

Keywords: maxillomandibular advancement, sleep quality, genioplasty, respiratory disturbance

1. Introduction

Obstructive sleep apnea (OSA) is a disorder characterized by intermittent and recurrent episodes of partial or complete upper airway obstruction during sleep. Obesity, a narrow nasopharynx and oropharynx, large soft palate, large tonsils, large tongue, tongue retroposition, micrognathia, mandibular retrognathia, and maxillary retrusion can all cause upper airway obstruction [1–8].

Maxillomandibular advancement (MMA) and genioglossus advancement (GA) improve airway volume, oxygen desaturation, and the apnea-hypopnea index (AHI) in patients with OSA. However, there are few reports on changes in sleep quality and architecture following MMA and GA [9]. Therefore, we assessed the effects of MMA and GA on sleep quality by comparing oxygen desaturation, AHI, and sleep architecture before and after MMA and GA.

2. Materials and methods

Nine OSA patients who had MMA and GA underwent polysomnography (PSG) before and after surgery, which was assessed using the same scoring criteria. One subject was excluded because computed tomography (CT) data were not collected, neither before nor after surgery. Our study included a total of eight subjects (six males and two females). The average age and body mass index (BMI) of the participants were 43.75 ± 8.17 years and 21.8 ± 1.8 kg/m2, respectively.

2.1 Surgical procedure

All patients underwent MMA using a standardized surgical procedure consisting of a LeFort I osteotomy and bilateral sagittal split ramus osteotomy and GA using a genioplasty to pull the genioglossus and geniohyoid muscles. The amount of maxillary advancement was routinely set at a minimum of 5 mm or more in consideration for unavoidable change in facial appearance. The mandibular jaw was advanced to match the maxilla, to restore the preoperative jaw relationship. The average amount of mandibular advancement was 13.2 mm. The average amount of skeletal advancement in GA was 6.3 mm. All patients were informed regarding the study protocol and provided consent.

2.2 Morphological evaluation

The lateral cephalometric radiograph were taken and calculated with manual hand-tracing.

The CT evaluation (1-mm slices) was performed with the aid of an Asteion device (TSX-021B/4; Toshiba, Tokyo, Japan), before and at 1 year after surgery. For standard reproducibility the patient was placed in the supine position, with the head and neck positioned on a pillow to maintain the Frankfurt plane at right angles to the floor. CT scans were performed during inspiration at rest, without swallowing. The upper airway area was measured in three regions: the superior posterior airway space (SPAS), which is the airway region at the midpoint between the inferior tip of the soft palate (P point) and the posterior nasal spine (PNS) point, parallel to the line from the gonion point to the point at the deepest midline concavity on the mandibular alveolus between the infradentale and pogonion (B point) (GO-B line); the middle airway space (MAS), which is the airway region on the P point parallel to the GO-B line; and the inferior airway space (IAS), which is the airway region on the GO-B line [10] (**Figures 1** and **2**).

The volume between PNS and Eb was also measured (**Figure 3**).

All data analyses were performed using Mimics software (Materialize, Leuven, Belgium).

2.3 Physiological evaluation (polysomnography)

Polysomnographic recordings were performed before and within 1 year after surgery. We used a 16-channel PSG instrument (Alice 5; Philips Respironics, Murrysville, PA, USA) with continuous monitoring performed by a technician.

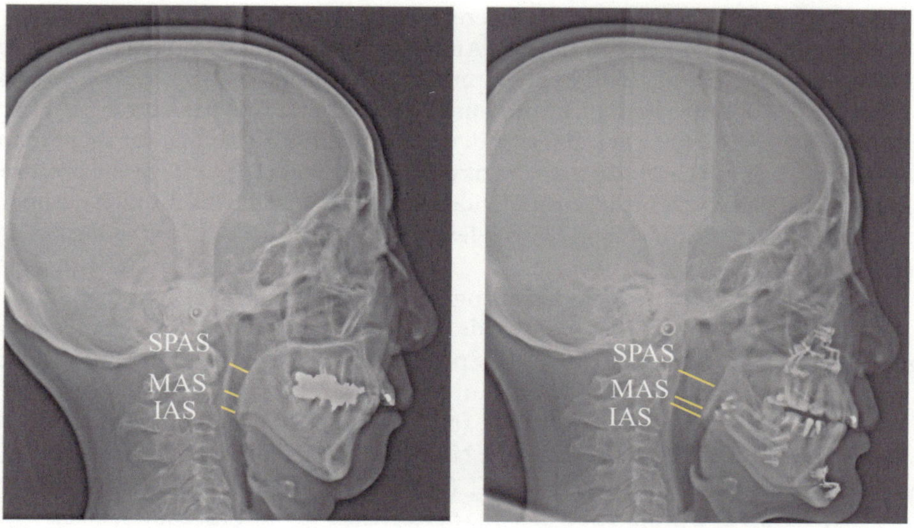

Figure 1.
Scheme of each of the measurement regions (anteroposterior dimension). SPAS, superior posterior airway space; MAS: Middle airway space; IAS: Inferior airway space.

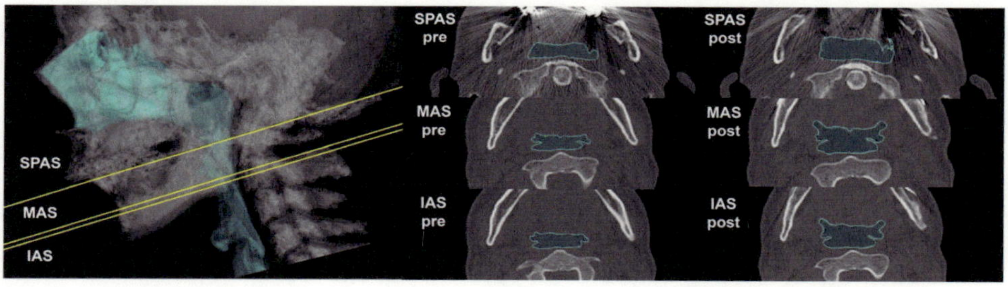

Figure 2.
Scheme of each of the measurement regions (cross-sectional area). SPAS, Superior posterior airway space; MAS, Middle airway space; IAS, Inferior airway space.

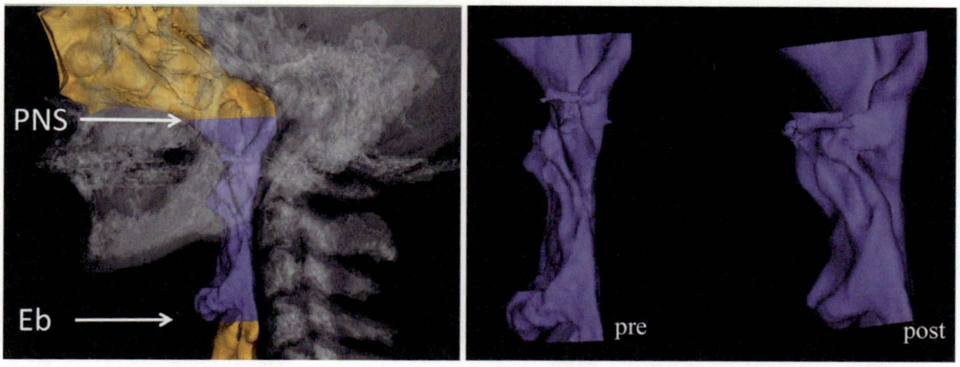

Figure 3.
Scheme of the measurement regions (volume). PNS, Posterior nasal spine; Eb, Epiglottal base.

The measures taken included electroencephalography (EEG), electrooculogram (EOG), electromyogram (EMG), electrocardiogram (ECG), snore, thermocouple airflow, nasal pressure, chest and abdominal movement, pulse oximetry, and body position. Polysomnographic analyses were performed according to the American Academy of Sleep Medicine guidelines. Apnea was defined as complete cessation of airflow for more than 10 seconds. Hypopnea was defined as a decrease in airflow of 90% or more from the baseline, as measured by an oronasal thermistor for at least 10 seconds, a 30% or greater reduction in respiratory airflow lasting for more than 10 seconds, or at least a 3% decrease in oxygen saturation (SpO_2) from the pre-event baseline. The 3% oxygen desaturation index (ODI) represents the average number of times per hour that the blood oxygen level drops by 3% from the baseline during sleep [9].

Arousal was defined as a sudden change in EEG frequency. We collected data on AHI, apnea index (AI), hypopnea index (HI), 3% ODI, lowest SpO_2, percentage at which SpO_2 was <90% of TST (%SpO_2 < 90%), total sleep time (TST), sleep efficiency (SE: TST/time in bed [TIB]), number of awakenings (NA), percentage of nonrapid eye movement sleep stage 1 (NREM1) of TST (%S1), percentage of NREM2 of TST (%S2), percentage of NREM3 of TST (%S3), percentage of rapid eye movement (REM) sleep of TST (%REM), wakefulness after sleep onset (WASO), WASO as a proportion of sleep period time (SPT) (%WASO), sleep latency, and REM latency.

All data were analyzed using the Wilcoxon t-test, with a value of $p < 0.05$ considered statistically significant.

3. Results

3.1 Change in the airway before versus after MMA and GA

The mean anteroposterior dimension of the SPAS, MAS, and IAS increased from 9.8 ± 3.24, 7.3 ± 2.93, and 9.6 ± 2.47 to 15.7 ± 3.67 ($p < 0.005$), 12.6 ± 2.94 ($p < 0.005$), and 15.4 ± 3.73 ($p < 0.005$), respectively (**Figure 4**).

The mean cross-sectional area of the SPAS, MAS, and IAS increased from 171.3 ± 104.6, 221.3 ± 66.6, and 200.9 ± 70.2 to 317.1 ± 141.7 ($p < 0.005$), 335.0 ± 132.8 ($p < 0.01$), and 316.9 ± 140.4 ($p < 0.01$), respectively. The mean enlargement factor of SPAS, MAS, and IAS was 213.0 ± 70.6%, 152.1 ± 47.3%, and 160.9 ± 54.8%, respectively. The mean volume between PNS and Eb increased from 13664.2 ± 5458.6 to 18647.0 ± 8456.0 ($p < 0.01$). The mean volume expansion rate was 136.5 ± 30.2% ($p < 0.01$) (**Figure 5**).

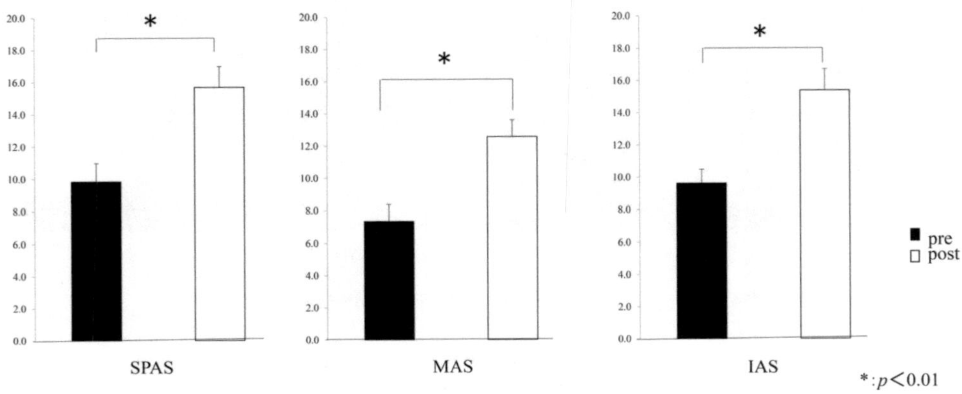

Figure 4.
Change in each anteroposterior dimension of airway before and after MMA and GA.

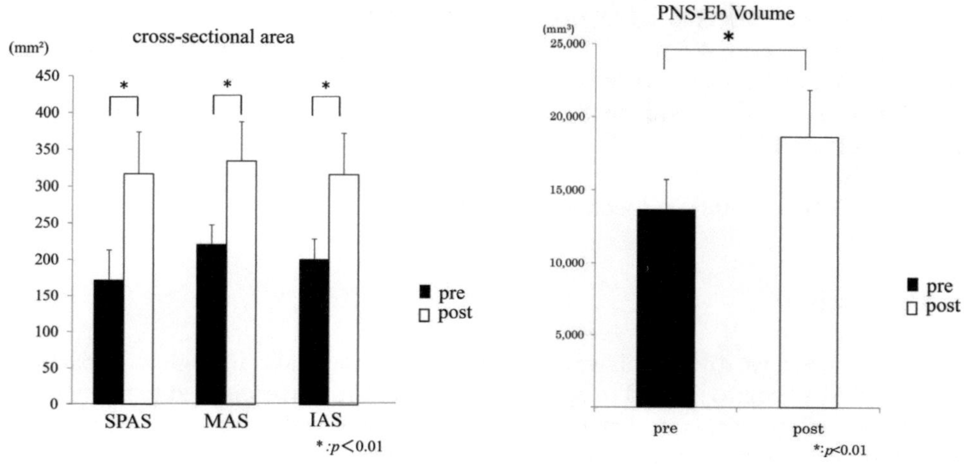

Figure 5.
Change in each cross-sectional area and volume of airway before and after MMA and GA.

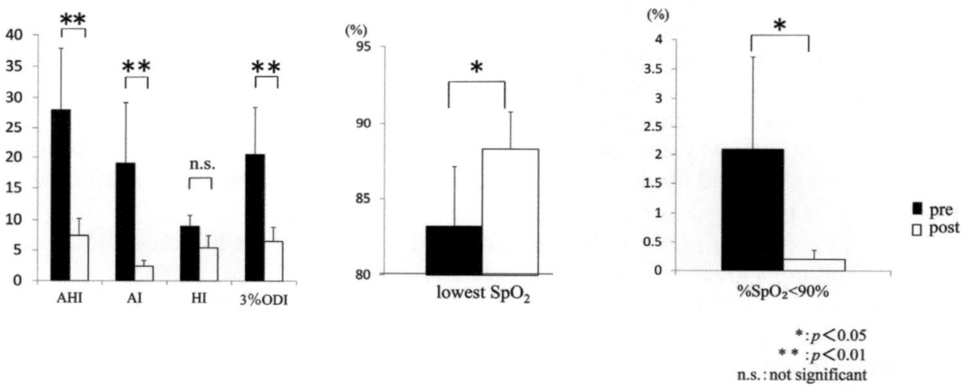

Figure 6.
Change in polysomnography parameter before and after MMA and GA (sleep-disordered breathing).

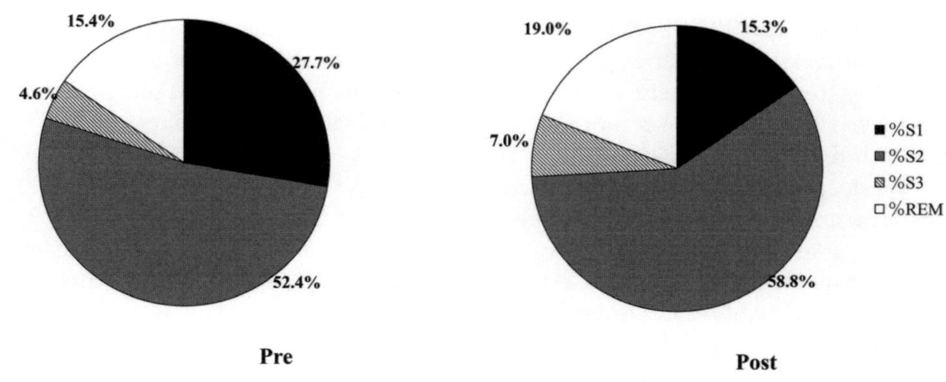

Figure 7.
Change in polysomnography parameter before and after MMA and GA (sleep stage).

3.2 Changes in PSG parameters in subjects before versus after MMA and GA

The mean AHI decreased from 28.0 ± 24.6 to 7.4 ± 6.9 events/hour ($p < 0.005$), the AI decreased from 19.0 ± 25.4 to 2.3 ± 2.4 ($p < 0.008$), the

ODI decreased from 20.5 ± 19.9 to 6.5 ± 5.9 ($p < 0.008$), and the %$SpO_2 < 90$% decreased from 2.1 ± 4.0 to 0.2 ± 0.4 ($p < 0.02$), while the mean lowest SpO_2 increased from 83.3 ± 9.5% to 88.3 ± 6.4% ($p < 0.02$) (**Figure 6**).

The mean SE increased from 81.2 ± 12.8 to 86.2 ± 7.7 ($p < 0.03$), and %REM increased from 15.4 ± 5.7% to 19.0 ± 3.6% ($p < 0.02$); meanwhile, the mean %S1 and NA decreased from 27.7 ± 21.2% to 15.3 ± 7.6% ($p < 0.01$) and 184.7 ± 108.4 to 119.5 ± 40.7 ($p < 0.008$), respectively (**Figure 7**).

4. Discussion

In this study, we divided airway space into retropalatal and retroglossal spaces: SPAS and MAS corresponded to retropalatal, while IAS corresponded to retroglossal. We found an increase in anteroposterior dimension and cross-sectional area of both the retropalatal and retroglossal spaces following MMA and GA, consistent with previous studies. The volume of airway space was also increased.

The retropalatal space is influenced by the position of the maxilla, soft palate, and tonsils, while the retroglossal space is influenced by the mandibular position and glossal shape and position [11–13]. The soft palate is comprised of the musculus uvulae, tensor veli palatini, levator veli palatini, and palatoglossus. The former three muscles are attached to the maxilla, while the latter is attached to the mandible. The genioglossus and geniohyoid muscles are attached to the mental spine and hyoid bone [14]. Airway enlargement is primarily caused by elevation of the tissues attached to the jaw and hyoid bone. Therefore, the most effective surgical approach to resolve this issue is to move both the upper and lower jaw.

Surgical success of MMA is defined as an AHI with less than 20 events/hour or an AHI showing a greater than 50% reduction after surgery. Meanwhile, surgical cure is defined as an AHI with less than five events/hour following surgery [15].

In this study, all patients were in the surgical success category, and 50% of patients were also classified as surgical cure.

The ODI and %$SpO_2 < 90$% both decreased, while the lowest SpO_2 increased; these results are consistent with previous reports [16]. These findings indicate that although achieving complete cure is difficult, MMA remains an effective method for treating sleep-disordered breathing. Furthermore, improvements in the lowest SpO_2 and %$SpO_2 < 90$% levels prevent the development of oxygen-desaturation-related diseases. A number of previous studies demonstrated that hypoxia-induced oxidative stress, sympathetic activation, and inflammatory responses increase the long-term risk of multiple comorbidities, including hypertension, heart attack, stroke, and diabetes [17–22].

The sleep architecture was also altered after MMA. There is currently no consensus on how “better sleep” should be quantitatively and qualitatively defined [9]. However, some researchers have suggested that decreased SE, TST, and percentage of slow-wave sleep (SWS) of TST (%SWS) and increased WASO are indicators of poor sleep quality [23–25]. Others believe that improved sleep quality is reflected by the increases in %REM and %SWS, based on prior CPAP treatment data [26]. Our study did not find any decrease in WASO. However, TST and %REM were both increased, while %S1 and NA both decreased. Furthermore, there is no significant difference, but SWS tends to increase. Based on these results, it appears that both the quality and quantity of sleep were improved.

OSA interrupts the normal sleep cycle: REM sleep disappears or becomes irregular, while SWS disappears. In our study, some subjects exhibited a REM pattern similar to that of healthy subjects, while in others no therapeutic effect of MMA was observed, despite sufficient airway expansion. Given the small number of subjects in our study, it was not possible to identify factors affecting the therapeutic efficacy. However, the most common causative factors of OSA include poor upper airway anatomy (collapsibility), weak upper airway dilator muscle responsiveness, a low respiratory arousal threshold, and an unstable ventilatory control system (loop gain) [27–30]. Taken together, we consider that oxygen inhalation and sleeping medication, for example, may prove therapeutic for patients with symptoms not improved by surgical intervention alone.

MMA and GA cannot provide equal effect for every patient. The airway expansion is affected by the amount of jaw movement. However, even if the airway expansion is made bigger, it does not necessarily improve the quality of sleep. So, I must further explore other factors involved in affecting sleep quality.

5. Conclusion

MMA and GA can increase the anteroposterior dimension, cross-sectional area, and volume of the retropalatal and retroglossal spaces, consistent with previous studies.

MMA and GA may be able to improve not only sleep respiratory disturbance but also improve sleep quality.

Acknowledgements

This study was supported by the Sato Fund, Nihon University School of Dentistry; a grant from the Dental Research Center, Nihon University School of Dentistry; and the Uemura Fund, Nihon University School of Dentistry.

Data herein have been previously applied to Nichidai Shigaku (in Japanese) by Ryota Nakamura.

Conflict of interest

The authors declare no conflict of interest.

Ethical approval

This study was performed with the approval of the Ethics Committee of Nihon University School of Dentistry.

Informed consent

Informed consent was obtained from all individual participants included in the study.

Author details

Takako Sato[1]*, Ryota Nakamura[1], Akio Himejima[1], Akemi Kusano[1], Serim Kang[1], Saori Ohtani[1], Kentarou Yamada[1], Kanako Yamagata[1], Hiroaki Azaki[1], Junya Aoki[1], Keiichi Yanagawa[1], Keiji Shinozuka[1], Takeya Yamada[2] and Morio Tonogi[1]

1 Department of Oral and Maxillofacial Surgery, Nihon University School of Dentistry, Tokyo, Japan

2 Hikone Municipal Hospital, Hikone, Japan

*Address all correspondence to: sato.takako@nihon-u.ac.jp

References

[1] Yagi H, Nakata S, Tsuge H, Yasuma F, Noda A, Morinaga M, et al. Morphological examination of upper airway in obstructive sleep apnea. Auris Nasus Larynx. 2009;**36**:444-449

[2] Hudgel DW, Hendricks C. Palate and hypopharynx—Sites of inspiratory narrowing of the upper airway during sleep. The American Review of Respiratory Disease. 1988;**138**:1542-1547

[3] Trudo FJ, Gefter WB, Welch KC, Gupta KB, Maislin G, Schwab RJ. State-related changes in upper airway caliber and surrounding soft-tissue structures in normal subjects. American Journal of Respiratory and Critical Care Medicine. 1998;**158**:1259-1270

[4] Zonato AI, Bittencourt LR, Martinho FL, Junior JF, Gregorio LC, Tufik S. Association of systematic head and neck physical examination with severity of obstructive sleep apnea–hypopnea syndrome. Laryngoscope. 2003;**113**:973-980

[5] Schellenberg JB, Maislin G, Schwab RJ. Physical findings and the risk for obstructive sleep apnea. The importance of oropharyngeal structures. American Journal of Respiratory and Critical Care Medicine. 2000;**162**:740-748

[6] Petrou-Amerikanou C, Belazi MA, Daskalopoulou E, Vlachoyiannis E, Daniilidou NV, Papanayiotou PC. Oral findings in patients with obstructive sleep apnea syndrome. Quintessence International. 2005;**36**:293-298

[7] Tsai WH, Remmers JE, Brant R, Flemons WW, Davies J, Macarthur C. A decision rule for diagnostic testing in obstructive sleep apnea. American Journal of Respiratory and Critical Care Medicine. 2003;**167**:1427-1432

[8] Riley RW, Powell N, Guilleminault C. Current surgical concepts for treating obstructive sleep apnea syndrome. Journal of Oral and Maxillofacial Surgery. 1987;**45**:149-157

[9] Liu SY-C, Huon L-K, Ruoff C, Riley RW, Strohl KP, Peng Z. Restoration of sleep architecture after maxillomandibular advancement: Pp beyond the apnea –hypopnea index. International Journal of Oral and Maxillofacial Surgery. 2017;**46**:1533-1538

[10] Furuhashi A, Yamada S, Shiomi T, Sasanabe R, Aoki Y, Yamada Y, et al. Effective three-dimensional evaluation analysis of upper airway form during oral appliance therapy in patients with obstructive sleep apnoea. Journal of Oral Rehabilitation. 2013;**40**:582-589

[11] Schendel SA, Broujerdi JA, Jacobson RL. Three-dimensional upper-airway changes with maxillomandibular advancement for obstructive sleep apnea treatment. American Journal of Orthodontics and Dentofacial Orthopedics. 2014;**146**(3):385-393

[12] Powell NB, Mihaescu M, Mylavarapu G, Weaver EM, Guilleminault C, Gutmark E. Patterns in pharyngeal airflow associated with sleep-disordered breathing. Sleep Medicine. 2011;**12**:966-974

[13] Stephen S, Powell N, Jacobson R. Maxillary, mandibular, and chin advancement: Treatment planning based on airway anatomy in obstructive sleep apnea. Journal of Oral and Maxillofacial Surgery. 2011;**69**:663-676

[14] Okushi T, Tonogi M, Arisaka T, Kobayashi S, Tsukamoto Y, Morishita H, et al. Effect of maxillomandibular advancement on morphology of velopharyngeal space. Journal of Oral and Maxillofacial Surgery. 2011;**69**:877-884

[15] Sher AE, Schechtman KB, Piccirillo JF. The efficacy of surgical modifications of the upper airway in adults with obstructive sleep apnea syndrome. Sleep. 1996;**19**:156-177

[16] Holty JE, Guilleminault C. Maxillomandibular advancement for the treatment of obstructive sleep apnea: A systematic review and meta-analysis. Sleep Medicine Reviews. 2010;**14**:287-297

[17] Vasu TS, Grewal R, Doghramji K. Obstructive sleep apnea syndrome and perioperative complications: A systematic review of the literature. Journal of Clinical Sleep Medicine. 2012;**8**:199-207

[18] Peppard PE, Young T, Palta M, Skatrud J. Prospective study of the association between sleep-disordered breathing and hypertension. The New England Journal of Medicine. 2000;**342**:1378-1384

[19] Tasali E, Mokhlesi B, Van Cauter E. Obstructive sleep apnea and type 2 diabetes: Interacting epidemics. Chest. 2008;**133**:496-506

[20] Sharma B, Owens R, Malhotra A. Sleep in congestive heart failure. The Medical Clinics of North America. 2010;**94**:447-464

[21] Yaggi HK, Concato J, Kernan WN, Lichtman JH, Brass LM, Mohsenin V. Obstructive sleep apnea as a risk factor for stroke and death. The New England Journal of Medicine. 2005;**353**:2034-2041

[22] Marin JM, Carrizo SJ, Vicente E, Agusti AG. Long-term cardiovascular outcomes in men with obstructive sleep apnoea-hypopnoea with or without treatment with continuous positive airway pressure: An observational study. Lancet. 2005;**365**:1046-1053

[23] Means MK, Edinger JD, Glenn DM, Fins AI. Accuracy of sleep perceptions among insomnia sufferers and normal sleepers. Sleep Medicine. 2003;**4**:285-296

[24] Coaters TJ, Killen JD, George J, Marchini E, Silverman S, Thoresen C. Estimating sleep parameters: A multitrait-multimethod analysis. Journal of Consulting and Clinical Psychology. 1982;**50**:345-352

[25] Perlis ML, Smith MT, Andrews PJ, Orff H, Giles DE. Beta/gamma EEG activity in patients with primary and secondary insomnia. Journal of Psychosomatic Research. 2009;**66**:59-65

[26] Riley RW, Powell NB, Guilleminault C. Maxillofacial surgery and nasal CPAP. A comparison of treatment for obstructive sleep apnea syndrome. Chest. 1990;**98**:1421-1425

[27] Eckert DJ, Owens RL, Kehlmann GB, Wellman A, Rahangdale S, Yim-Yeh S, et al. Eszopiclone increases the respiratory arousal threshold and lowers the apnoea/hypopnoea index in obstructive sleep apnoea patients with a low arousal threshold. Clinical Science (London). 2011;**120**:505-514

[28] Heinzer RC, White DP, Jordan AS, Lo YL, Dover L, Stevenson K, et al. Trazodone increases arousal threshold in obstructive sleep apnea. The European Respiratory Journal. 2008;**31**:1308-1312

[29] Wellman A, Malhotra A, Jordan AS, Stevenson KE, Gautam S, White DP. Effect of oxygen in obstructive sleep apnea: Role of loop gain. Respiratory Physiology & Neurobiology. 2008;**162**:144-151

[30] Edwards BA, Sands SA, Eckert DJ, White DP, Butler JP, Owens RL, et al. Acetazolamide improves loop gain but not the other physiological traits causing obstructive sleep apnoea. The Journal of Physiology. 2012;**590**:1199-1211

Chapter 10

Body Dysmorphic Disorder in Oral and Maxillofacial Surgery

Türker Yücesoy

Abstract

Body dysmorphic disorder (BDD) may be related to the appearance of a body part or may sometimes arise from concerns about a body function. Currently, this disorder was included in contemporary classification systems with DSM-5. The majority of BDD patients first consult dermatologists, surgeons, and more often plastic surgeons, rather than psychiatrists. Therefore, it is difficult to determine the prevalence of this disorder in the psychiatric society. The oral and maxillofacial region is highly associated with face deformities, and the patients with BDD are applying to those clinics even without self-awareness of their disorders. It has been reported that most of the orthognathic surgical patients are associated with the facial appearance of surgical motivations and will have similar psychological motivations to cosmetic surgery patients. Moreover, the orthodontics, prosthetic and restorative dentistry are the branches of dentistry that mostly the patients come with esthetic complaints. Studies on BDD have not yet received the value they deserve concerning the prevalence and severity. Researches in dentistry and oral and maxillofacial surgery are much less, and the individuals suffering from BDD are not well-known among dentists/oral and maxillofacial surgeons; therefore, the frequency of BDD patients is not noticed and treated properly.

Keywords: body dysmorphic disorder, maxillofacial surgery, esthetics, dentistry, psychiatry

1. Description

Most people are not completely satisfied with their appearance. But some individuals are very concerned about a slight or imaginary flaw in their appearance. These individuals could have a "problem" not only physically but also psychiatrically.

Body dysmorphic disorder (BDD) is a condition not only in which a person overestimates and exaggerates a body defect but also one may believe in the existence even if there is not a body defect. This engagement can lead to significant unrest or impaired functionality. BDD is a severe illness and relatively common which often presents to both mental health professionals and nonpsychiatric physicians [1].

1.1 History

The disorder was defined as "compulsive neurosis" in the first place. After, it was called "obsession with shame of the body" and "dysmorphophobia," respectively. Dysmorphophobia is preferred to explain the sudden emergence and continuation of the idea of a deformity; it is defined as an individual's fear of the occurrence of this deformity and feeling the anxiety of this awareness considerably [2].

Body dysmorphic disorder was first shown in the DSM-IV in 1980 and described as an atypical somatoform disorder [3]. The American Psychiatric Association (APA) classified this "problem" as a distinct somatoform disorder in 1987, and since then it has gained popularity in the media and in clinical researches [4]. Currently, BDD is included in contemporary classification systems with DSM-5 (the *Diagnostic and Statistical Manual of Mental Disorders, 5th Edition*), the classification system of the APA [5].

1.2 Diagnosis

The changes between DSM 4 and DSM 5 criteria for diagnosing BDD are shown in **Figure 1**. On the other hand, many tests have been established to diagnose BDD or measure its severity. However, some tests are performed more frequently for specific reasons, such as easy application and providing more effective results, for example, the Body Image Disturbance Questionnaire (BIDQ) [6], Yale-Brown Obsessive–Compulsive Scale Modified for BDD (BDD-YBOCS) and Body Dysmorphic Disorder Questionnaire (BDDQ) [7], the Cosmetic Procedure Screening (COPS) questionnaire [8], the Appearance Anxiety Inventory (AAI) [9], BDD Dimensional Scale (BDD-D) [10], the Body Image Disturbance Questionnaire (BIQLI) [11], and the Dysmorphic Concern Questionnaire (DCQ) [12].

1.3 Epidemiology

BDD is a relatively common disorder. Despite its prevalence and severity, the diagnosis can be missed in clinical settings [13]. The majority of BDD patients first consult dermatologists, internists, surgeons, and more often plastic surgeons, rather than psychiatrists. Therefore, it is difficult to determine the prevalence of this disorder in the psychiatric society. Although the studies in the general population range from 0.7 to 5.3% [14–18], clinical studies reveal higher rates: 8.8 to 12% [19, 20] among dermatology patients; 7% in cosmetic surgery patients [21]; 14–42% in patients with atypical major depression [22–24]; 11–13% in patients with social anxiety [25, 26]; 8–37% in patients with obsessive–compulsive disorder [26–28]; and 39% in patients with anorexia nervosa [29].

DSM-IV	DSM-5
Disorder Class: Somatoform Disorders	Disorder Class: Obsessive-Compulsive and Related Disorders
A. Preoccupation with an imagined defect in appearance. If a slight physical anomaly is present, the person's concern is markedly excessive.	A. Preoccupation with one or more perceived defects or flaws in physical appearance that are not observable or appear slight to others.
	B. At some point during the course of the disorder, the individual has performed repetitive behaviors (e.g., mirror checking, excessive grooming, skin picking, reassurance seeking) or mental acts (e.g., comparing his or her appearance with that of others) in response to the appearance concerns.
B. The preoccupation causes clinically significant distress or impairment in social, occupational, or other important areas of functioning.	C. The preoccupation causes clinically significant distress or impairment in social, occupational or other areas of functioning.
C. The preoccupation is not better accounted for by another mental disorder (e.g., dissatisfaction with body shape and size in anorexia nervosa).	D. The appearance preoccupation is not better explained by concerns with body fat or weight in an individual whose symptoms meet diagnostic criteria for an eating disorder.
--	*Specify* if: With muscle dysmorphia: The individual is preoccupied with the idea that his or her body build is too small or insufficiently muscular. This specifier is used even if the individual is preoccupied with other body areas, which is often the case. *Specify* if: Indicate degree of insight regarding body dysmorphic disorder beliefs (e.g., "I look ugly" or "I look deformed"). With good or fair insight: The individual recognizes that the body dysmorphic disorder beliefs are definitely or probably not true or that they may or may not be true. With poor insight: The individual thinks that the body dysmorphic beliefs are probably true. With absent insight/delusional beliefs: The individual is completely convinced that the body dysmorphic beliefs are true.

Figure 1.
DSM-IV to DSM-V body dysmorphic disorder comparison.

Despite the presence of BDD cases beginning in adulthood or childhood, symptoms often begin in adolescence or young adulthood [30]. In particular, men and young people do not want to report their complaints because of humiliation and embarrassment or do not see them as a mental problem. Although the age of onset goes down to 6 years, in many studies the age of onset is reported to be between the ages of 15 and 20, with an average age of 16–18 [31].

1.4 Quality of life and functionality

The main cognitive feature of BDD is the belief that extreme anxiety and imagined defect represent a personal disability. One's quality of life can vary considerably. Many people can at least limit their social functions and resort to avoidance in order to prevent their imperfections from appearing fully in the public sphere. These avoidance strategies may include camouflage by wearing makeup or concealed clothing. Some individuals may never leave the house. Phillips et al. reported that men with BDD had a higher rate of single or single living than women, whereas another study found that 30% of BDD patients were individuals who could not leave their homes at least 1 week before the study [32, 33]. Other compulsive behaviors are to examine, heal, or conceal the perceived defects and include excessive mirror control, excessive care, styling hair, camouflaging the defect, comparing oneself with others, picking skin, and trying to convince the ugliness of the defect to others [34]. Therefore, psychosocial functioning of BDD is associated with suicidal tendencies and especially poor quality of life [35].

1.5 Classification

Although BDD was classified as a somatoform disorder in DSM-IV, it is currently accepted as a disorder of the obsessive–compulsive spectrum disorders (OCSD) group because of its overlapping aspects with OCSD in DSM-V. However, it is frequently emphasized that BDD not only is a clinical variant of OCSD but is also associated with mood disorders, social anxiety disorders, and eating disorders [36].

1.6 Clinical symptoms

The main clinical features of BDD are disproportionately dealing with an imaginary or mild physical defect, which leads to significant clinical distress or a significant loss of functionality in work, private, and social life. It is known that most patients with BDD do not consult with psychiatrists and apply to nonpsychiatric physicians, such as esthetic surgeons, to eliminate the perceived physical defects. Sixty eight to ninety-eight percent of BDD patients experience concerns about multiple body regions [32, 37].

BDD may be related to the appearance of a body part or may sometimes arise from concerns about a body function. Sweating and related thoughts about the secretion of bad odor can be given as an example. Concerns of BDD cases become more apparent in social settings. Avoidance behaviors such as being unable to go out of the house or going out in the dark only, not being able to enter social environments due to concerns, and leaving school or work are common symptoms. Most of the patients believe that their physical defects are seen and noticed by others, and therefore they look at the mirror in excessive levels or try to stay away from the objects that reflect the mirror image as much as possible, make use of makeup material, and make dress changes in order to hide the areas that they believe to be defective.

1.7 Co-diagnosis

The most common comorbid diagnoses in BDD are major depression, social phobia, drug addictions, and OCD [38]. Phillips et al. showed that the frequency of OCD was 37% among 100 cases [39], and similarly the incidence of OCD was found to be 39% of the study of 50 cases by Hollander et al. [37].

1.8 Differential diagnosis

Because BDD and OCD have similar features in many respects, BDD is often accepted as an OCD [40–42]. However, poorer insight than OCD, higher suicide rates, and higher comorbidity of depression differentiate the two disorders [41, 43, 44]. A significant proportion of patients diagnosed with BDD show avoidance behaviors in social settings. This situation evokes the avoidance behaviors of social phobic patients [43]. Social phobia cases are comfortable as long as they stay away from crowded environments that cause anxiety for them.

Social phobia patients also know that their concerns are meaningless, but they cannot resist their anxiety. While individuals with BDD do not think their concerns are meaningless, staying away from social settings does not reduce the anxiety of such patients. Also, in social phobia, the reason for staying away from the social environment is not usually exaggerated physical defects [13, 35].

1.9 Treatment

Many individuals with BDD resort to nonpsychiatric medical and surgical treatments to correct perceived defects in their physical appearance. Dermatological treatment is the most desirable and applied treatment (mostly acne agents). It is followed by surgical treatment, most commonly rhinoplasty. In a study in which 12% of subjects received isotretinoin, treatment rarely increased BDD. Therefore, nonpsychiatric medical treatments do not seem to be effective in the treatment of body dysmorphic disorder. Crerand et al. stated that individuals were also evaluated, and the results reported that individuals who refused psychiatric treatment did not observe any change and their condition worsened [45]. The somatic subtype of delusional disorder needs to be distinguished from BDD. The somatic subtype of delusional disorder provides more benefits than antipsychotic medication; BDD patients benefit from treatment with selective serotonin reuptake inhibitors (SSRIs) [38, 41]. The general opinion is that the use of high-dose SSRIs in BDD will be beneficial [46, 47]. The use of SSRI is considered to be the ideal treatment when the highest dose recommended by the manufacturer for 12 weeks or more is used. Daily fluvoxamine 150 mg, fluoxetine 40 mg, paroxetine 40 mg, sertraline 150 mg, citalopram 40 mg, and escitalopram 20 mg SSRI doses are considered as the minimum and adequate doses [48]. Any treatment of "defect" in patients with BDD is controversial. However, the general idea is that surgical treatments should be performed if only these individuals still need surgery after psychiatric treatment [49].

1.10 Translation of the scales and questionnaires

Due to almost all the scales being prepared in English, the translation of those forms into other languages and validity and reliability studies should be performed, and it must be proven that it is equivalent to the original language. For example, the translation of the YBOCS-BDD scale into Brazilian Portuguese was performed among 93 selected rhinoplasty patients of both sexes. Also, the test–retest method was used for reliability at 1-week intervals, and statistical analysis was performed using correlation coefficient and intraclass correlation coefficient (ICC) [50]. It has also been translated into Persian, German, French, and Italian, and these studies have shown significant results [51, 52]. In the German reliability and validity study of the BIDQ-S scale, which is a modification of the BIDQ scale for scoliosis patients, 259 patients with idiopathic scoliosis were included in the study [53].

2. Body dysmorphic disorder in oral and maxillofacial surgery

The developed scales have been mentioned in many studies in the world, including esthetics such as dermatology, esthetic surgery, maxillofacial surgery, and orthodontics, and have been used to detect individuals with BDD (**Figure 2**). But the maxillofacial region is highly associated with face deformities, and the patients with BDD are applying to those clinics even without self-awareness of their disorders. Particularly, orthognathic surgery, also known as corrective jaw surgery, is considered functional surgery in the treatment of maxillomandibular dysfunction. However, the correction of maxillomandibular deformity creates highly esthetic and satisfactory results. In the studies in the literature, it has been reported that 52–74% of orthognathic surgical patients are associated with the facial appearance of surgical motivations and will have similar psychological motivations to cosmetic surgery patients. After this type of surgery, satisfaction with the outcome is as high as 92%, resulting in improved quality of life [54–56]. In a small number of patients (<10%) who are not satisfied with the surgical outcome, the underlying cause may be a psychological condition experienced by the individual rather than a failed surgical procedure. The underlying psychological condition may be BDD, which is believed to be increased in patients seeking orthognathic surgery [56]. It was found that 10% of orthognathic surgery patients met significantly higher BDD criteria than reported rates (between 0.7 and 4.0%) in the general adult population [15, 57–59]. This rate is similar to the prevalence of cosmetic surgery and dermatology patient population of BDD, which is between 6 and 16% [60].

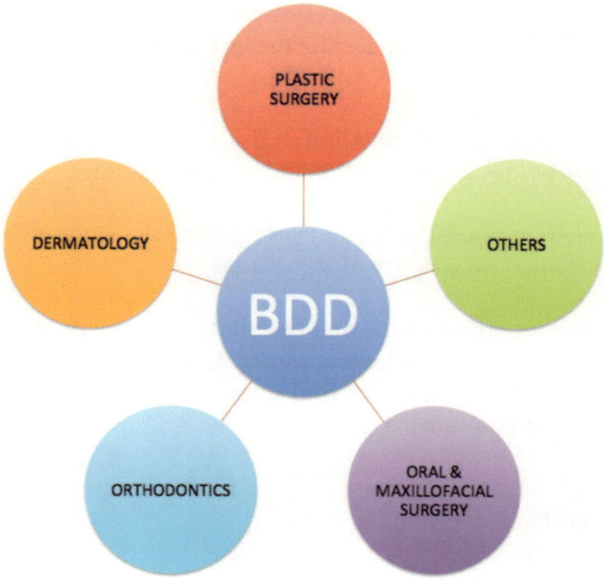

Figure 2.
Nonpsychiatric departments where body dysmorphic disorder patients generally apply to.

Although researches on BDD and dental treatment are relatively rare, published case reports showed the BDD patients involved in general dentistry and maxillofacial surgery. Some authors applied a questionnaire to 40 adult patients who participated in orthodontic treatment and estimated the prevalence of BDD to be 7.5%, suggesting that individuals with BDD had a high demand for orthodontic treatment [34]. De Jongh et al. reported the frequency of occupation of individuals with a defect in their appearance and stated that the rate of whitening and orthodontic treatment of those who reported that they were engaged in such defect was nine times higher [60]. These studies have shown that clinicians working in esthetic dentistry are likely to be visited by BDD patients and therefore need to be aware of the condition of such patients and to know how to evaluate and manage patients suspected of having BDD [49].

In addition to areas such as plastic surgery and dermatology, another important part where the patient comes with esthetic complaints is dentistry. Maxillofacial surgery, orthodontics, prosthetic, and restorative dental treatment, which is a branch of dentistry, are among the important parts that patients come with esthetic complaints. The inability to detect individuals with possible BDD in these departments and to try to eliminate the esthetic complaint before the treatment of psychiatric disorder adversely affects the success of the treatment.

Eventually, all of those studies show that the prevalence of BDD among dentist individuals is much more severe than the general population. Moreover, the incidence of BDD patients among individuals who apply to clinics is unknown. To increase the success rate of the treatment by increasing the satisfaction rate obtained as a result of the esthetic treatments, further studies should be planned to identify the individuals with BDD. The importance of informing the patients preoperatively in dentistry/maxillofacial surgery must be well-known. The studies should aim to increase the frequency of application of the tests for BDD in dentistry to determine the real epidemiology of this disease among this field.

3. Conclusion

- The patients with BDD apply to all clinics to relieve their esthetic concerns which are the main complaint despite the lack of self-awareness of the psychological disorder.

- These clinics may be dental, maxillofacial surgery, dermatology, and esthetic surgery that provide esthetic treatment to a large extent.

- Worldwide research on BDD has not yet received the value it deserves concerning the prevalence and severity of the disease.

- Researches in dentistry and oral and maxillofacial surgery are much less than in other departments. Individuals suffering from BDD are not well-known among dentists/oral and maxillofacial surgeons; therefore, the frequency of BDD patients is not noticed.

Conflict of interest

None.

Author details

Türker Yücesoy
Department of Oral and Maxillofacial Surgery, Faculty of Dentistry, Bezmialem Vakif University, Istanbul, Turkey

*Address all correspondence to: dt.yucesoy@hotmail.com

References

[1] Phillips KA. The presentation of body dysmorphic disorder in medical settings. Primary Psychiatry. 2006;**13**(7):51

[2] Fava GA. Morselli's Legacyi: Dysmorphophobia. Psychotherapy and Psychosomatics. 1992;**58**(3-4):117-118

[3] Crerand CE, Franklin ME, Sarwer DB. Body dysmorphic disorder and cosmetic surgery. Plastic and Reconstructive Surgery. 2006;**118**(7):167e-180e

[4] Hunt TJ, Thienhaus O, Ellwood A. The mirror lies: Body dysmorphic disorder. American Family Physician. 2008;**78**(2):217-224

[5] American Psychiatric Association. Diagnostic and statistical manual of mental disorders (DSM-5®). USA: American Psychiatric Publishing; 2013

[6] Cash TF, Phillips KA, Santos MT, Hrabosky JI. Measuring "negative body image": Validation of the body image disturbance questionnaire in a nonclinical population. Body Image. 2004;**1**(4):363-372

[7] Phillips KA, Hollander E, Rasmussen SA, Aronowitz BR. A severity rating scale for body dysmorphic disorder: Development, reliability, and validity of a modified version of the Yale-Brown obsessive compulsive scale. Psychopharmacology Bulletin. 1997;**33**(1):17

[8] Veale D, Ellison N, Werner TG, Dodhia R, Serfaty M, Clarke A. Development of a cosmetic procedure screening questionnaire (COPS) for body dysmorphic disorder. Journal of Plastic, Reconstructive & Aesthetic Surgery. 2012;**65**(4):530-532

[9] Veale D, Eshkevari E, Kanakam N, Ellison N, Costa A, Werner T. The appearance anxiety inventory: Validation of a process measure in the treatment of body dysmorphic disorder. Behavioural and Cognitive Psychotherapy. 2014;**42**(5):605-616

[10] LeBeau RT, Mischel ER, Simpson HB, Mataix-Cols D, Phillips KA, Stein DJ, et al. Preliminary assessment of obsessive–compulsive spectrum disorder scales for DSM-5. Journal of Obsessive-Compulsive and Related Disorders. 2013;**2**(2):114-118

[11] Hrabosky JI, Cash TF, Veale D, Neziroglu F, Soll EA, Garner DM, et al. Multidimensional body image comparisons among patients with eating disorders, body dysmorphic disorder, and clinical controls: A multisite study. Body Image. 2009;**6**(3):155-163

[12] Mancuso SG, Knoesen NP, Castle DJ. The Dysmorphic concern questionnaire: A screening measure for body dysmorphic disorder. The Australian and New Zealand Journal of Psychiatry. 2010;**44**(6):535-542

[13] Bjornsson AS, Didie ER, Phillips KA. Body dysmorphic disorder. Dialogues in Clinical Neuroscience. 2010;**12**(2):221

[14] Bienvenu OJ, Samuels JF, Riddle MA, Hoehn-Saric R, Liang K-Y, Cullen BA, et al. The relationship of obsessive–compulsive disorder to possible spectrum disorders: Results from a family study. Biological Psychiatry. 2000;**48**(4):287-293

[15] Bohne A, Keuthen NJ, Wilhelm S, Deckersbach T, Jenike MA. Prevalence of symptoms of body dysmorphic disorder and its correlates: A cross-cultural comparison. Psychosomatics. 2002;**43**(6):486-490

[16] Cansever A, Uzun Ö, Dönmez E, Özşahin A. The prevalence and clinical

features of body dysmorphic disorder in college students: A study in a Turkish sample. Comprehensive Psychiatry. 2003;**44**(1):60-64

[17] Faravelli C, Salvatori S, Galassi F, Aiazzi L, Drei C, Cabras P. Epidemiology of somatoform disorders: A community survey in Florence. Social Psychiatry and Psychiatric Epidemiology. 1997;**32**(1):24-29

[18] Sarwer DB, Cash TF, Magee L, Williams EF, Thompson JK, Roehrig M, et al. Female college students and cosmetic surgery: An investigation of experiences, attitudes, and body image. Plastic and Reconstructive Surgery. 2005;**115**(3):931-938

[19] Phillips KA, Dufresne RG Jr, Wilkel CS, Vittorio CC. Rate of body dysmorphic disorder in dermatology patients. Journal of the American Academy of Dermatology. 2000;**42**(3):436-441

[20] Uzun Ö, Başoğlu C, Akar A, Cansever A, Özşahin A, Çetin M, et al. Body dysmorphic disorder in patients with acne. Comprehensive Psychiatry. 2003;**44**(5):415-419

[21] Sarwer DB, Wadden TA, Pertschuk MJ, Whitaker LA. Body image dissatisfaction and body dysmorphic disorder in 100 cosmetic surgery patients. Plastic and Reconstructive Surgery. 1998;**101**(6):1644-1649

[22] Nierenberg AA, Phillips KA, Petersen TJ, Kelly KE, Alpert JE, Worthington JJ, et al. Body dysmorphic disorder in outpatients with major depression. Journal of Affective Disorders. 2002;**69**(1-3):141-148

[23] Perugi G, Akiskal H, Lattanzi L, Cecconi D, Mastrocinque C, Patronelli A, et al. The high prevalence of "soft" bipolar (II) features in atypical depression. Comprehensive Psychiatry. 1998;**39**(2):63-71

[24] Phillips KA, Nierenberg AA, Brendel G, Fava M. Prevalence and clinical features of body dysmorphic disorder in atypical major depression. The Journal of Nervous and Mental Disease. 1996;**184**(2):125-129

[25] Brawman-Mintzer O, Lydiard RB, Phillips KA, Morton A, Czepowicz V, Emmanuel N, et al. Body dysmorphic disorder in patients with anxiety disorders and major depression: A comorbidity study. The American Journal of Psychiatry. 1995;**152**(11):1665-1667. Available from: https://doi.org/10.1176/ajp.152.11.1665

[26] Wilhelm S, Otto MW, Zucker BG, Pollack MH. Prevalence of body dysmorphic disorder in patients with anxiety disorders. Journal of Anxiety Disorders. 1997;**11**(5):499-502

[27] Pigott TA, L'Heureux F, Dubbert B, Bernstein S, Murphy DL. Obsessive compulsive disorder: comorbid conditions. The Journal of Clinical Psychiatry. 1994;**55**:15-27. discussion 28-32

[28] Simeon D, Hollander E, Stein DJ, Cohen L, Aronowitz B. Body dysmorphic disorder in the DSM-IV field trial for obsessive-compulsive disorder. The American Journal of Psychiatry. 1995;**152**(8):1207-1209

[29] Grant JE, Kim SW, Eckert ED. Body dysmorphic disorder in patients with anorexia nervosa: Prevalence, clinical features, and delusionality of body image. International Journal of Eating Disorders. 2002;**32**(3):291-300

[30] Hollander E, Aronowitz BR. Comorbid social anxiety and body dysmorphic disorder: Managing the complicated patient. The Journal of Clinical Psychiatry. 1999;**60**:27-31

[31] Veale D, Boocock A, Gournay K, Dryden W, Shah F, Willson R, et al. Body dysmorphic disorder: A survey

of fifty cases. The British Journal of Psychiatry. 1996;**169**(2):196-201

[32] Phillips KA, McElroy SL, Keck PE, Pope HG, Hudson JI. Body dysmorphic disorder: 30 cases of imagined ugliness. American Journal of Psychiatry. 1993;**150**:302-302

[33] Phillips KA, Menard W, Fay C. Gender similarities and differences in 200 individuals with body dysmorphic disorder. Comprehensive Psychiatry. 2006;**47**(2):77-87

[34] Hepburn S, Cunningham S. Body dysmorphic disorder in adult orthodontic patients. American Journal of Orthodontics and Dentofacial Orthopedics. 2006;**130**(5):569-574

[35] Phillips K. In: Phillips KA, editor. Body Dysmorphic Disorder, in Somatoform and Factitious Disorders. Washington, DC: American Psychiatric Press; 2001

[36] Castle DJ, Rossell SL. An update on body dysmorphic disorder. Current Opinion in Psychiatry. 2006;**19**(1):74-78

[37] Hollander E, Cohen LJ, Simeon D. Body dysmorphic disorder. Psychiatric Annals. 1993;**23**(7):359-364

[38] Gunstad J, Phillips KA. Axis I comorbidity in body dysmorphic disorder. Comprehensive Psychiatry. 2003;**44**(4):270-276

[39] Phillips KA, McElroy SL, Keck PE, Hudson JI, Pope H. A comparison of delusional and nondelusional body dysmorphic disorder in 100 cases. Psychopharmacology Bulletin. 1994;**30**(2):179-186

[40] Cohen LJ, Stein DJ, Simeon D. Obsessive-compulsive spectrum disorders. In: Hollander E, Stein DJ, editors. Obsessive-Compulsive Disorders. New York: Marcel Dekker Inc; 1997. pp. 47-74

[41] Phillips KA, Gunderson CG, Mallya G, McElroy SL, Carter W. A comparison study of body dysmorphic disorder and obsessive-compulsive disorder. The Journal of Clinical Psychiatry. 1998;**59**(11):568-575

[42] Frare F, Perugi G, Ruffolo G, Toni C. Obsessive–compulsive disorder and body dysmorphic disorder: A comparison of clinical features. European Psychiatry. 2004;**19**(5):292-298

[43] Buhlmann U, Wilhelm S, McNally RJ, Tuschen-Caffier B, Baer L, Jenike MA. Interpretive biases for ambiguous information in body dysmorphic disorder. CNS Spectrums. 2002;7(6):435-443

[44] Eisen JL, Phillips KA, Coles ME, Rasmussen SA. Insight in obsessive compulsive disorder and body dysmorphic disorder. Comprehensive Psychiatry. 2004;**45**(1):10-15

[45] Crerand CE, Phillips KA, Menard W, Fay C. Nonpsychiatric medical treatment of body dysmorphic disorder. Psychosomatics. 2005;**46**(6):549-555

[46] Phillips KA. The Broken Mirror: Understanding and Treating Body Dysmorphic Disorder. USA: Oxford University Press; 2005

[47] Phillips KA. Understanding Body Dysmorphic Disorder. USA: Oxford University Press; 2009

[48] Ray PÇ, Demirkol ME, Tamam L. Beden dismorfik bozukluğu. Psikiyatride Güncel Yaklaşımlar. 2012;**4**(4):547-565

[49] Cunningham S, Bryant C, Manisali M, Hunt N, Feinmann C. Dysmorphophobia: Recent developments of interest to the maxillofacial surgeon. British Journal of Oral and Maxillofacial Surgery. 1996;**34**(5):368-374

[50] MJd B, Sabino Neto M, de Oliveira MF, Cordás TA, Duarte LS, Rosella MF, et al. Yale-Brown obsessive compulsive scale modified for body dysmorphic disorder (BDD-YBOCS): Brazilian Portuguese translation, cultural adaptation and validation. Brazilian Journal of Psychiatry. 2015;**37**(4):310-316

[51] Rabiee M, Khorramdel K, Kalantari M, Molavi H. Factor structure, validity and reliability of the modified Yale-brown obsessive compulsive scale for body dysmorphic disorder in students. Iranian Journal of Psychiatry and Clinical Psychology. 2010;**15**(4):343-350

[52] Rush AJ Jr, First MB, Blacker D. Handbook of Psychiatric Measures. USA: American Psychiatric Publishing; 2009

[53] Wetterkamp M, Thielsch MT, Gosheger G, Boertz P, Terheyden JH, Schulte TL. German validation of the BIDQ-S questionnaire on body image disturbance in idiopathic scoliosis. European Spine Journal. 2017;**26**(2):309-315

[54] Cheng L, Roles D, Telfer M. Orthognathic surgery: The patients' perspective. British Journal of Oral and Maxillofacial Surgery. 1998;**36**(4):261-263

[55] Espeland L, Høgevold HE, Stenvik A. A 3-year patient-centred follow-up of 516 consecutively treated orthognathic surgery patients. The European Journal of Orthodontics. 2007;**30**(1):24-30

[56] Olson R, Laskin D. Expectations of patients from orthognathic surgery. Journal of Oral Surgery. 1980;**38**(4):283-285

[57] Buhlmann U, Glaesmer H, Mewes R, Fama JM, Wilhelm S, Brähler E, et al. Updates on the prevalence of body dysmorphic disorder: A population-based survey. Psychiatry Research. 2010;**178**(1):171-175

[58] Koran LM, Abujaoude E, Large MD, Serpe RT. The prevalence of body dysmorphic disorder in the United States adult population. CNS Spectrums. 2008;**13**(4):316-322

[59] Otto MW, Wilhelm S, Cohen LS, Harlow BL. Prevalence of body dysmorphic disorder in a community sample of women. American Journal of Psychiatry. 2001;**158**(12):2061-2063

[60] De Jongh A, Oosterink F, Van Rood Y, Aartman I. Preoccupation with one's appearance: A motivating factor for cosmetic dental treatment? British Dental Journal. 2008;**204**(12):691

Chapter 11

Psychosocial and Health-Related Quality of Life (HRQoL) Aspect of Oral and Maxillofacial Trauma

Ramat Oyebunmi Braimah, Dominic Ignatius Ukpong and Kizito Chioma Ndukwe

Abstract

Psychosocial and health-related quality of life following oral and maxillofacial injuries is an often neglected aspect of patients' management. It has been noted that patients with maxillofacial trauma were more likely to be depressed, anxious with low self-esteem and poor health-related quality of life and possibility of post-traumatic stress disorder (PTSD). Depression and anxiety associated with facial trauma are often coupled with worries regarding recovery. Following trauma, there may be physical dysfunction especially facial disfigurement which may adversely affect the patients' ability to undertake daily activities and lower their mood and self-esteem leading to overall poor health-related quality of life. Focusing on these psychosocial factors, this chapter also elaborated on the immediate and long term effects of these factors if not incorporated into patient's care. In a study of 80 maxillofacial injured patients' in Sub-Saharan Africa using hospital anxiety and depression scale (HADS) questionnaire, the HADS detected 42 (52.5%) cases of depression and 56 (70.0%) cases of anxiety at baseline. Rosenberg's self-esteem questionnaire detected 33 (41.3%) patients with low self-esteem at baseline. WHO HRQoL-Bref questionnaire showed poor Quality of life in all the domains of the instrument with lowest in the physical and psychological domains. Similarly, the trauma screening questionnaire (TSQ) for PTSD detected 19 patients had symptoms of PTSD at Time 1 with a prevalence rate of 25%.

Keywords: anxiety, depression, injury, maxillofacial, self-esteem, quality of life, post-traumatic stress disorder

1. Introduction

Following maxillofacial trauma, the psychosomatic requirements of patients are distinctive and very important. Studies have shown that individuals with maxillofacial trauma often presents with signs of depression/sadness, worry/anxiety and aggression/hostility over 1 year period after such traumatic conditions as compared to equaled control group [1]. Similarly, several authors have documented that 10–70% of maxillofacial trauma patients showed signs of sadness and worry [1]. Often, these patients have other psychosocial troubles such as joblessness, illiteracy and poor societal support [2]. Many times these symptoms are sub-threshold and might not meet the diagnostic benchmarks for a psychiatric condition. Subsequently, these subthreshold symptoms often lead to problem-solving dilemmas, deprived management of the condition and poor interventions. Other symptoms that may complicate the dilemma include normative reactions to sadness, anguish over the losses in such trauma, complications from medications and exhaustion from treatment.

Depression puts the individual at more danger of suicidal tendencies, reduced treatment compliance, and poor convalescence aftermath. In such cases, quality of life and recovery from the maxillofacial trauma are often compromised [3, 4].

1.1 Psychosocial morbidity of patients with facial trauma

Although maxillofacial fractures are one of the more common types of injuries, studies frequently publish epidemiology of maxillofacial injuries and management protocol. Such studies only from surgical management tend to disregard salient symptoms that can impact health aftermaths.

Throughout the preceding decade, the efforts of some investigators [5–7] have increasingly sensitized the surgical community to the hidden social and psychological factors that adversely influence treatment response and increase the risk of re-injury. Through the efforts of these investigators, maxillofacial injuries are now seen and managed both surgically and psychologically [8]. Although, efficient surgical repair is a critical aspect of recuperation, meeting the psycho-social needs that may put them at specific risk for poor psychological adjustment is equally important after the traumatic incident.

When these emotional and behavioral disorders, including depression and antisocial behavior remains untreated, it leads to deprived social performance, job-related fiasco, drug and substance abuse that upsurges the peril of violence and re-injury [5]. Based on these facts, the current mode of management should be a multidisciplinary approach wherein surgeons and other specialists (psychologists, psychotherapists and psychiatrists) will formulate a treatment plan that would addresses the surgical and psychosocial needs following maxillofacial trauma [5, 9].

1.1.1 Depression and anxiety

Depression and anxiety related with maxillofacial injuries are often linked with concerns regarding recovery and stretch of the treatment course [10]. Disfigurement often associated with maxillofacial trauma also affects the social image of the individual with such injuries [11]. Social withdrawal and isolation is major sequelae that may ensue following the facial disfigurement with feeling inferior and social stigmatization [12, 13]. Many times recovery from maxillofacial injuries is often protracted with multiple surgeries and complex postoperative management to restore function. This protracted course may add to patient's frustration [14].

Injuries to vital regions of the face such as the eyes, ears, and dental hard tissue injuries often increase exposure to stress and hinder recovery [15]. Substantial difficulties in returning to premorbid levels of work-related functioning have also been noted in these cases [16]. Maxillofacial trauma patients also report higher rates of somatoform symptoms, drug abuse, PTSD symptoms, body aura issues, stigmatization, lesser quality of life, and lower overall contentment with life [17]. Also, maxillofacial trauma patients report snags in marital, work-related, and social functioning [18, 19].

1.1.2 Self-esteem

In psychology, self-esteem is a term used to echo a person's overall emotional evaluation of his or her own worth. Self-esteem is the level, to which one respects, values, accepts, admires, and likes oneself [20]. During the mid-1960s, Rosenberg, a social learning theorist, defined self-esteem as a personal worth or worthiness [20].

The significance of self-esteem lies in the fact that it concerns one's self, the way we are and the sense of our personal worth. Thus, self-esteem affects the way we are, the way we act in the world, and the way we relate with everyone else [21]. Furthermore, the way individuals reflect, feels, decides, and act is swayed by self-esteem. Low self-esteem is having a generally damaging overall outlook of oneself, judging or evaluating oneself negatively, and placing a general deleterious value on oneself as a person [21]. Low self-esteem can also have an impact on many aspects of a person's life. It can affect a person's functioning at work or at school. People with low self-esteem might not participate in many relaxation or entertaining activities, as they might believe that they do not justify any pleasure or fun [21]. Individual self-care could also be affected and might drink alcohol heavily and also abuse drugs and substances [21].

1.1.3 Health-related quality of life (HRQoL)

In everyday life, facial appearance plays an important function and roles. The appearance and "attractiveness" of an individual to one another is partially contributed by the person's face [22]. Following maxillofacial trauma, the individual may suffer facial defacement, chronic facial pain, anosmia, dysosmia, speech, dental, and ocular infirmities. Often times, concern is dedicated on the apparent physical aspect of maxillofacial trauma while the impact on the patient's psychological makeup and quality of life (QoL) is relegated to the background or even ignored. Most of the studies on psychological consequences and QoL in patients following maxillofacial injuries have been conducted in Western countries. Such studies in Sub-Saharan Africa and Middle East are rare [23].

1.1.4 Post-traumatic stress disorder

Other interesting and possible sequelae of trauma are post-traumatic stress disorder (PTSD). This disorder starts with an initial event of the trauma, which causes the person to feel intense fear, helplessness, and horror. The event is re-experienced either during the daytime in the form of distressing flashbacks or at night as terrifying dreams. This again causes fear, dread and a heightened state of psychological arousal in which patient tends to restrict activities and constrict thoughts and emotions in an effort to avoid re-experiencing the trauma. This disorder significantly distresses the individual and is highly associated with marital, occupational, financial and health problems [24–27]. Several investigators have reported PTSD rates of between 27 and 41% after maxillofacial injuries majorly caused by assault and interpersonal violence [1, 28], however, a preliminary Nigerian study reported a rate of 17.4% after maxillofacial trauma majorly caused by motorcycle accidents [23].

1.2 Psychological philosophies for the maxillofacial surgeon

When managing patients with maxillofacial injuries, the psychosocial aspect of the management must follow some general principles and must be kept in mind during reconstructive surgeries [29]. All efforts must be geared toward creating some realistic expectations for both patients and their families regarding surgical upshot. The duration to complete reconstruction, possible total number of surgeries, and degree of life disruptions and pain that may likely occur should be clearly explained to both patients and relatives [29]. One of the most significant roles that the handling surgeon can make is to take time to thoroughly listen to the victims and relatives' unique worries concerning the surgery, its sequel, and their capability living with defacement [30].

While many surgical team will satisfactorily respond to the psychological wants of their patients, many will require little additional psychosocial care like creating extra time, devotion and encouragement [31]. However, if the surgical team felt the patient and family may be assisted further by interrelating with psychiatrist or psychologists, such consultation should be expedited immediately by the surgical team.

Over the years, there has been some advancement made in focusing on the specific psychosocial worries of persons with maxillofacial disfigurement, including addressing the need for social skills improvement. Application of cognitive-behavioral forms which have been proven to very valuable will assist patients to cope with persistent negative social response following disfigurement from trauma. Furthermore, developing and spreading effective psycho-educational materials will also address specific concerns for those living with facial disfigurement [32].

2. Investigation of psychosocial and health-related quality of life after maxillofacial trauma

The authors carried out a research to investigate the psychological and health-related quality of life among maxillofacial injured patients in Sub-Saharan Africa (Nigeria). This was a prospective repeated measure designed to evaluate psychological characteristics and health-related quality of life in subjects with maxillofacial trauma who presented at the Oral/Maxillofacial Surgery Unit or Accident & Emergency Unit, Obafemi Awolowo University Teaching Hospital Complex, Ile-Ife, Nigeria.

2.1 Methodology

The study population was consecutive subjects with maxillofacial injuries attending the Accident and Emergency Unit or Oral/Maxillofacial Surgery Unit of the Obafemi Awolowo University Teaching Hospital Complex Ile-Ife Nigeria. Participants were recruited over a period of 12 months after approval from the hospital's Ethics and Research Committee. Adult subjects above 18 years irrespective of sex, race and type of injury were recruited after informed consent for the study was given. Additionally, they satisfied all the specified inclusion criteria. Head injured patients were excluded. Baseline interview was conducted within 1 week of arrival in the hospital (Time 1). Follow-up interviews were conducted at intervals of 4–8 weeks after initial contact (Time 2) and 10–12 weeks thereafter (Time 3).

2.2 Instruments for data collection

2.2.1 Demographics and clinical data collection

Data such as age, sex, level of education, occupation, and marital status was stored with questionnaire specially designed for such. The clinical data retrieved included cause of injury, location of injury, category of injury, and whether treatment was open reduction with internal fixation or closed reduction. Information about use of alcohol, drugs and other psychoactive substances were also obtained and recorded.

2.2.2 Hospital anxiety and depression scale (HADS)

This is a 14-item self-reporting tool with anxiety and depression subscales [33]. Each detail is rated on a four-point gradation, with each subscale having a range of 0–21. The HADS data collection instrument has been authorized in Nigerian hospitals and community samples [34]. The endorsed cut-off mark of seven for this region was adopted for this study [34].

2.2.3 Rosenbergs self-esteem questionnaire

This is a screening instrument for self-esteem [20]. The scale is a 10 item statement. Retrieved scores were calculated as follows:

- For questions 1, 2, 4, 6 and 7: They are rated as follows: strongly agree = 3, agree = 2, disagree = 1, strongly disagree = 0.

- For items 3, 5, 8, 9 and 10 (which are upturned in valence): They are rated as follows: strongly agree = 0, agree = 1, disagree = 2, strongly disagree = 3.

The scale ranged from 0 to 30. Marks between 15 and 25 are within normal range while marks below 15 insinuate low self-esteem. The Rosenberg self-esteem scale has been used in earlier research in Nigeria [35].

2.2.4 Quality of life (QoL)

World Health Organization QoL assessment instrument 26-item (WHO QoL-Bref) was used in assessing the QoL of individuals with maxillofacial injuries. This brief version QoL is a generic measure designed for use within a broad range of psychological and physical disorders [36]. It is a multidimensional tool, and was established for cross-cultural use; it assesses personal QoL. It comprises 26 queries and uses a five-point interval Likert response scale. For our study, the four domain model was applied. The four domains are those of physical health, psychological health, social relationships, and environment. Scores for domains were transformed on a scale of 4–20, with 20 being the highest and four being the lowest (see **Table 1** for steps in checking, cleaning data and computing domain scores for WHO QoL-Bref and also manual for converting raw scores to transformed scores). Scores were scaled in a positive direction. Higher scores denote high QoL and low scores shows low QoL. The WHO QoL-Bref has been widely used in Nigeria [37].

2.2.5 Post-traumatic stress disorder (PTSD)

The Trauma Screening Questionnaire [38] (TSQ) is a brief 10-item self-report measure devised to screen for posttraumatic stress disorder (PTSD). Each item is copied from the DSM-IV [25] criteria and describes either a re-experiencing symptom of PTSD (items 1–5) or a provocation symptom of PTSD (items 6–10). Evading and numbing symptoms, though also listed in the DSM-IV criteria, were not included in the TSQ in keeping with the authors' goal of creating a useful screening tool that was "short and contained the least amount of items essential for precise case identification" [38]. The TSQ has been able to predict excellent levels of PTSD following preliminary psychometric data [38] from two samples (rail crash survivors and crime victims). The principal author states that "what the TSQ gains in simplicity and clarity more than compensates for the absence of symptoms that may be difficult to understand and judgments that may be difficult to make" [39]. The authors have

DOMAIN 1		
Raw Score	Trasnformed scores	
	4-20	0-100
7	4	0
8	5	6
9	5	6
10	6	13
11	6	13
12	7	19
13	7	19
14	8	25
15	9	31
16	9	31
17	10	38
18	10	38
19	11	44
20	11	44
21	12	50
22	13	56
23	13	56
24	14	63
25	14	63
26	15	69
27	15	69
28	16	75
29	17	81
30	17	81
31	18	88
32	18	88
33	19	94
34	19	94
35	20	100

DOMAIN 2		
Raw score	Trasnformed scores	
	4-20	0-100
6	4	0
7	5	6
8	5	6
9	6	13
10	7	19
11	7	19
12	8	25
13	9	31
14	9	31
15	10	38
16	11	44
17	11	44
18	12	50
19	13	56
20	13	56
21	14	63
22	15	69
23	15	69
24	16	75
25	17	81
26	17	81
27	18	88
28	19	94
29	19	94
30	20	100

DOMAIN 3		
Raw score	Transformed scores	
	4-20	0-100
3	4	0
4	5	6
5	7	19
6	8	25
7	9	31
8	11	44
9	12	50
10	13	56
11	15	69
12	16	75
13	17	81
14	19	94
15	20	100

DOMAIN 4		
Raw score	Transformed scores	
	4-20	0-100
8	4	0
9	5	6
10	5	6
11	6	13
12	6	13
13	7	19
14	7	19
15	8	25
16	8	25
17	9	31
18	9	31
19	10	38
20	10	38
21	11	44
22	11	44
23	12	50
24	12	50
25	13	56
26	13	56
27	14	63
28	14	63
29	15	69
30	15	69
31	16	75
32	16	75
33	17	81
34	17	81
35	18	88
36	18	88
37	19	94
38	19	94
39	20	100
40	20	100

Table 1.
Manual for converting raw scores to transformed scores.

suggested administering the TSQ at least 3 weeks after the traumatic event "to allow for natural recovery processes." An ideal cut-off point was found to be a YES response to *at least* six re-experiencing or arousal symptom items, in any combination.

2.2.6 Statistical analysis

Data was analyzed with SPSS version 16 (SPSS 16 Inc., Chicago, IL, USA). Results were calculated as frequencies (%), means and standard deviations (SD) for normally distributed variables.

3. Results presentation

3.1 Socio-demographics

The study population consisted of 80 participants. There were 64 (80.0%) males and 16 (20.0%) females. The mean age of the sample was 33.2 ± 12.5, range 18–70 years. Road traffic accidents were responsible for a sizeable proportion of injuries in the facial injured (68 (85%)). The socio-demographic characteristics of the study population are shown in **Tables 2** and **3**. Only 21 patients where admitted and most of them were discharged home within 1 week of hospital stay (16 (76.2%)) as shown in **Table 4**.

	Facial injury (%)
Sex	
Male	64 (80.0)
Female	16 (20.0)
Age	
Young adult (18–35)	60 (75.0)
Middle age (36–44)	10 (12.5)
Elderly (45–70)	10 (12.5)
Marital status	
Married	47 (58.8)
Single	33 (41.2)
Divorced	0 (0.0)
Education	
No education	2 (2.5)
Primary	13 (16.2)
Secondary	41 (51.3)
Tertiary	24 (30)
Occupation	
Unemployed	21 (26.3)
Unskilled	30 (37.5)
Skilled	14 (17.5)
Professional	12 (15.0)
#Others	3 (3.7)
Type of house	
Personal	15 (18.8)
Rented	64 (80.0)
No house	1 (1.2)
Admission	
Yes	21 (26.3)
No	59 (73.7)

#*Voluntary workers.*

Table 2.
Socio-demographic characteristics.

	Facial injury (%)
Complex PTSD	
Assault	6 (7.5)
Road traffic accident	68 (85.0)
Others (fall and occupational injury)	6 (7.5)
Type of RTA	
Motorcycle	52 (76.6)
Car	9 (13.2)
Truck	1 (1.4)
Bus	6 (8.8)
Combined	0 (0.0)
Road location	
Intercity	26 (37.7)
Intracity	43 (62.3)
Status of patient	
Driver	43 (64.2)
Passenger	24 (35.8)
Pedestrian	0 (0.0)
Vehicle factor	
Burst tyre	9 (25.0)
Failed brakes	0 (0.0)
Unknown	27 (75.0)
Driver factor	
Over speeding	30 (68.2)
Drunk	2 (4.5)
Slept off	0 (0.0)
Unknown	12 (27.3)

Table 3.
Sociodemographic characteristics (continued).

Duration of hospital stay (week)	Facial injury (n = 21) (%)
<1	16 (76.2)
4–8	5 (23.8)
10–12	—
>12	—
Total	21 (100)

Table 4.
Distribution of duration of hospital stay and injury.

Mandibular fracture was the most frequently fractured facial bone (n = 46) followed by mandible + maxillary fracture (n = 14). The distribution of these is shown in **Table 5** and **Figure 1**. Fifty-two (65%) of the facial injured patients had soft tissue injuries in addition to their facial bone fractures.

Sixty-seven subjects (83.8%) were managed with closed reduction of the fractured bone, 13 (16.2%) were treated with open reduction and rigid internal fixation (**Table 6**).

3.2 Anxiety and depression

3.2.1 Anxiety

The Hospital anxiety and Depression scale (HADS) detected 56 (70.0%) had anxiety at baseline, 32 (42.1%) at Time 2 and only 9 (11.8%) had anxiety at Time 3. There was reduction in anxiety levels with time with only 9 (11.8%) having anxiety after 10–12 weeks post trauma (**Table 7**).

Type	Right (%)	Left (%)	#Combined (%)	Total (%)
Mandible	12 (26.1)	16 (34.8)	18 (39.1)	46 (100)
Maxilla	4 (36.4)	1 (9.1)	6 (54.5)	11 (100)
Zygomatic bone	7 (100)	0	0	7 (100)
Mandible + maxilla	3 (21.4)	3 (21.4)	8 (57.2)	14 (100)
Maxilla + zygomatic	0	0	2 (100)	2 (100)
Total				80 (100)

#Combined (both right and left).

Table 5.
Distribution of facial bone fracture.

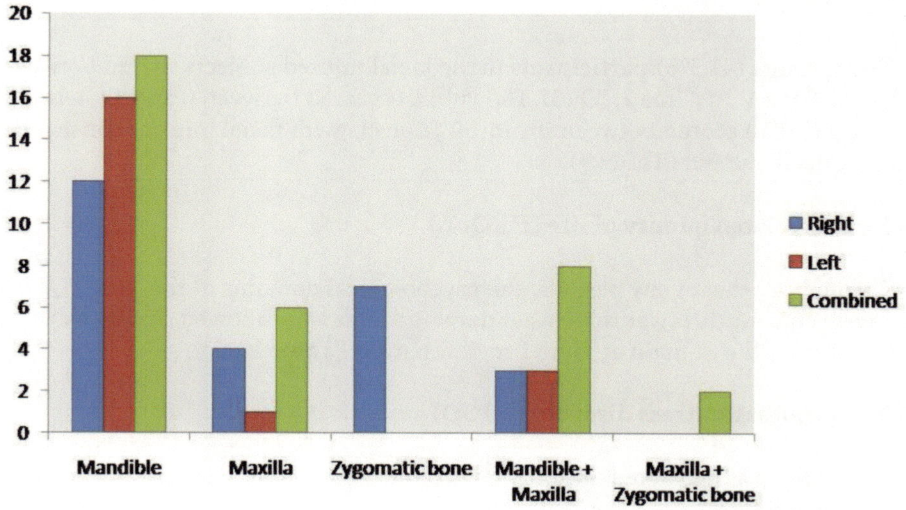

Figure 1.
Bar chart showing distribution of maxillofacial bone fractures.

Type of treatment	Facial injury (%)
Closed reduction	67 (83.8)
Open reduction	13 (16.2)
Total	80 (100)

Table 6.
Distribution of types of treatment received by the facial fracture.

Time	Facial injury
Time 1 (within 1 week of injury)	(n = 80)
	10.8 (3.3)
	56 (70.0%)[#]
Time 2 (4–8 weeks)	(n = 76)
	6.5 (3.2)
	32 (42.1%)[#]
Time 3 (10–12 weeks)	(n = 76)
	3.9 (3.1)
	9 (11.8%)[#]

[#]*Proportion of subjects with high anxiety scores.*

Table 7.
Change in mean HADS anxiety scores (M ± SD) with time.

3.2.2 Depression

The Hospital anxiety and Depression scale (HADS) detected 42 (52.5%) cases of depression at baseline, 36 (47.4%) cases at Time 2 and 14 (18.4%) cases at Time 3 (These are subjects that scored above the cut-off point of 7 on the Depression scale of the HADS). There was reduction in depression levels with time (**Table 8**).

3.3 Self-esteem

Thirty-three (41.3%) participants in the facial injured subjects scored between 0 and 14 at Time 1. At Time 2, 39 (51.3%) subjects scored between 0 and 14, while at Time 3, 7 (9.2%) scored between 0 and 14. Subjects with facial injuries consistently had lower self-esteem (**Table 9**).

3.4 Health-related quality of life (HRQoL)

Throughout the review periods, the psychological domains of the WHO QoL-Bref were constantly lower than other domains. This was followed closely by the social relationship domain at Time 1 review period (**Table 10**).

3.5 Post-traumatic stress disorder (PTSD)

The PTSD was evaluated only at Times 2 and 3 consistent with the commencement of evaluation after 3 weeks of injury. Seventy-six patients were screened out of the 80 participants at Times 1 and 2. Nineteen patients had symptoms of PTSD at Time 1 and 20 patients at Time 2 with a prevalence rates of 25.0 and 26.3% respectively (**Figure 2**).

Time	Facial injury
Time 1 (within 1 week of injury)	(*n* = 80)
	8.4 (3.4)
	42 (52.5%)#
Time 2 (4–8 weeks)	(*n* = 76)
	7.4 (2.5)
	36 (47.4%)#
Time 3 (10–12 weeks)	(*n* = 76)
	6.4 (1.7)
	14 (18.4%)#

#*Proportion of subjects with high depression score.*

Table 8.
Change in mean HADS depression scores (M ± SD) with time.

Time	Facial injury
Time 1 (within 1 week of injury)	(*n* = 80)
#Score 0–14	33 (41.3%)
¶Score 15–30	47 (58.7%)
Time 2 (4–8 weeks)	(*n* = 76)
#Score 0–14	39 (51.3%)
¶Score 15–30	37 (48.7%)
Time 3 (10–12 weeks)	(*n* = 76)
#Score 0–14	7 (9.2%)
¶Score 15–30	69 (90.8%)

#*Low self-esteem.*
¶*Normal self-esteem.*

Table 9.
Changes in proportion of subjects with low and normal self-esteem with time.

Domains at Times 1, 2, and 3	Facial injury
Time 1 (1 week or less)	
Physical health	11.0 (±1.8)
Psychological health	9.3 (±1.8)
Social relationship	10.5 (±2.6)
Environment	11.4 (±2.3)
At Time 2 (4–8 weeks)	
Physical health	12.5 (±1.5)
Psychological health	11.4 (±1.8)
Social relationship	13.1 (±2.5)
Environment	12.9 (±1.6)
At Time 3 (10–12 weeks)	
Physical health	13.5 (±1.3)
Psychological health	12.9 (±1.8)
Social relationship	15.8 (±6.7)
Environment	14.3 (±2.5)

Table 10.
Change in mean WHO (HRQoL-Bref) score according to domains at Times 1, 2, and 3.

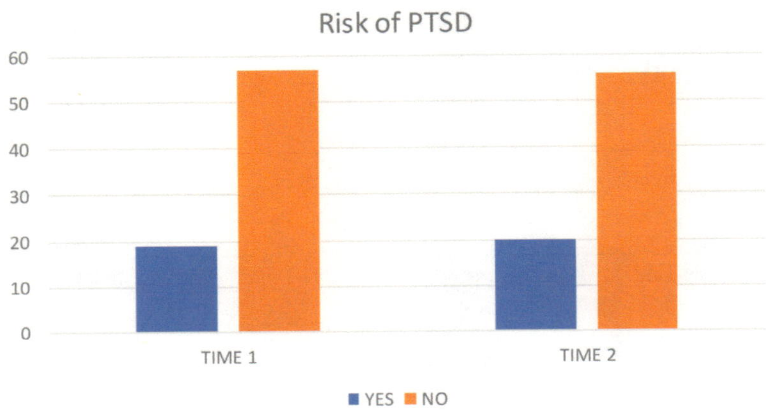

Figure 2.
Bar chart showing distribution of number of maxillofacial injured having potential for post-traumatic stress disorder (PTSD) at Times 1 and 2.

4. Discussion

4.1 Socio-demographics

The management of maxillofacial is largely driven by the obvious clinical manifestations of the physical injury, while the less evident psychosocial sequelae are rarely considered [40]. Documented possible symptoms of these psychological sequelae following facial trauma include increase in levels of depression, anxiety, phobic anxiety, and obsessive compulsive tendencies [40]. The appearance and "attractiveness" of a person to other people is partly contributed by the person's face. As a result of maxillofacial trauma, the patient may suffer facial disfigurement.

Previous reports [23, 41–43] have supported these new findings where 84% of injuries resulted from road traffic accidents. Road traffic accident continue to account for the most common reason of maxillofacial injury because of insufficient vehicular maintenance, lack of traffic laws enforcement, and poor levels of educational status of drivers [44]. In United Kingdom, United States of America and other parts of the world, the mandatory uses of seat belts, crash helmets, traffic law enforcement, and increase in use of vehicles with airbags have reduced the incidence of maxillofacial injuries due to road traffic accident [45, 46].

Majority of the road traffic accident were motorcycle related, 76.6% in facial injured subjects. This is because motorcycle is still a major means of transportation in Sub-Saharan Africa and riders do not often wear protective helmets making them more prone to head and facial injuries. Frequent traffic congestion because of poor road maintenance/network has made this mode of transportation attractive in most communities because motorcycles can navigate through narrow ways [44]. Whereas motorcycle-related facial trauma has been on the increase in Nigeria, a study in Europe however showed a decline in the incidence of such injuries in motorcycle-related accident [47]. Enforcement and use of appropriate crash helmets, increasing vehicle ownership due to increase in wealth were the reasons given for this decrease.

Assault-related maxillofacial injuries remain the main cause of maxillofacial trauma in industrialized nations [28, 48, 49]. This was not observed in this study as assault accounted for only 6 (7.5%) cases of facial trauma.

The present study recorded male preponderance. The reason for this observation is that motorcycle operators were predominantly males [34]. This pattern is in agreement with previous findings were male preponderance was reported [42, 43, 48].

The overall mean age for the study population was 33.2 (SD ± 12.5) years. This finding is also in agreement with previous studies where young adults are frequently involved in road traffic accidents [43, 50]. This age group is the period of high activity and individuals in this age group are more likely to take part in dangerous and risky exercises and sports, drive motor vehicle and motorcycles carelessly and are likely to be involved in violence [51]. More than half of the subjects who sustained injuries were either unemployed or involved in unskilled jobs. These findings echoed previous findings that patients with maxillofacial injuries have psychosocial problems like anxiety and depression, low self-esteem, unemployment, lower educational level and poor social support [2].

4.2 Anxiety and depression

The maxillofacial injured subjects were anxious from this study. This is comparable to previous reports of high rate of psychosocial complication following maxillofacial trauma [1, 28]. This present findings contrast those of previous study in south west Nigeria [23] where researchers stated that 11.8% of individuals sustaining maxillofacial injuries faced extreme anxiety levels immediately after injury, 3.0% during 4–8 weeks and 13.0% at 10–12 weeks follow-up times. While both studies were carried out in a comparable setting, the reason for the disparity could not be described; however, the authors opined that higher attrition rate in the earlier study might be responsible.

This study has shown high levels of depression in maxillofacial injured subjects. The findings are similar to those of previous researches investigating psychosocial complications of traumatic injury [1, 23, 28, 52]. A comparable finding in an erstwhile Nigerian study stated that 41.2% of patients had depression at Time 1 (within 10 days of injury), 47.1% at Time 2 (6–8 weeks after injury), and 21.7% at Time 3 (10–12 weeks after injury) [23]. This similarity was because both studies were carried out in similar study population and environment. The etiology of injury was also similar. Higher proportion of maxillofacial facial injured patients were depressed at Times 2 and 3 (47.4 and 18.4%, respectively) from previous study. This pattern is possibly as 52 (65%) patients of the maxillofacial injured sustained concomitant maxillofacial soft tissue wounds with the additional enduring scarring that could not be masked. This long-lasting scarring may alter their form and personality leading to social retraction and loss of self-esteem [16]. In addition, disfiguring might be the etiology of constant depression and be a continuous reminder of the mishap or act of violence where the injury occurred [53]. Though, the anxiety and depression levels were decreasing over the review times, it did not totally cease. Lento et al. [40] have described comparable outcomes whereby notwithstanding the decline in signs of psychological grief over time, additional psychological snags were still reported in injured group than the comparison cohort.

Other reports [40, 54] have opined that post-traumatic symptomatology may be an extension of earlier psychosocial problems and these individuals may be inadequately equipped psychologically to endure the pressures of the injury and recovery. Prior psychological status of persons in the third world nations is not a usual practice, therefore background psychological position of our patients were unavailable.

Extensive literature search yielded only two published data on risks of anxiety and depression following maxillofacial trauma from Sub-Saharan Africa [23, 55]. Additionally, our outcomes reverberated the need for reconstructive surgeons and other healthcare professionals to identify these psychosocial agonies together with the physical injuries sustained by these patients. Also, trauma care givers must be informed and trained in offering brief psychologic evaluations.

4.3 Self-esteem

The human face is the central point of identity of a person, and the existence of scar may alter a person's identity, which could lead to seclusion and loss of self-esteem. Additionally, when such injuries affect functions like speech and feeding, a maxillofacial injured subject may develop psychosocial problems [15, 56, 57]. Studies has also acknowledged the fact that nice-looking persons are more likely to have better self-esteem, accomplish higher levels of educational and job-related satisfaction, have more satisfying sexual encounters, and will generally have a better quality of life [58]. Consequently, it is rational to resolve that living with a maxillofacial defacement puts the person at an increased peril of undergoing a drastically reduced low quality of life and low self-esteem [2].

Psychological interventions are needed in the near aftermath of trauma in maxillofacial injured, as esteem needs of victims are frequently compromised. In this study, patients who screened positive for low self-esteem were referred to the psychiatry unit of the hospital for further follow-up. The strongest deficits in self-esteem were seen in the 1st week after injury and again from 6 to 8 weeks during recovery. This showed that maxillofacial injured consistently had low self-esteem throughout the review periods [59].

4.4 Health-related quality of life

Lower HRQoL after physical trauma has been reported in other studies [60]. In addition, it is probable that the physical dysfunction caused by these injuries may adversely affect the patients' ability to undertake their daily activities like tooth brushing, eating which will lower their mood and sense of self-esteem [60]. From the study, it will be observed that throughout the review periods, the psychological domains of the WHO QoL-Bref were constantly lower than other domains. This shows that maxillofacial injured are psychologically affected apart from the physical injuries they sustained. Similarly, the social relationship domain at Time 1 review period was also lower than other domains. Social relationships after maxillofacial injuries was also affected whereby patient may abstain from social interactions due to presence of scars on the face or inability to speak especially following intermaxillary fixation [61].

4.5 Post-traumatic stress disorder (PTSD)

Maxillofacial trauma may occur in life-threatening situations and as a result of accidents or industrial mishaps [62]. This may often herald the onset of PTSD. The principal symptoms of PTSD comprise (i) re-experiencing of the incidence (e.g., having unpleasant and upsetting thoughts and/or distressing images and dreams); (ii) evasion of thoughts, emotions or situations linked to the incidence; and (iii) autonomic nervous system hyperarousal, including struggles with sleeping, having an exaggerated disconcert response and undergoing increased irritability and nervousness [63].

From the current study, 19 patients had symptoms of PTSD at Time 1 and 20 patients at Time 2 with a prevalence rates of 25.0% and 26.3% respectively. This shows that in African population, there is high risk of patients with maxillofacial injuries to developing PTSD. A previous preliminary Nigerian study have reported a rate of 17.4% after maxillofacial trauma majorly caused by motorcycle accidents [23]. The current study showed a higher prevalence rate probably due to lower attrition rate as compared to previous study which reported a high attrition rate.

Studies have shown that there is the proof of PTSD signs and symptoms in adult acquired maxillofacial trauma patients [1, 28]. Similarly, it is likely that a significant lot of patients might experience sub-clinical forms of PTSD (i.e., not meeting the full diagnostic benchmarks) that can greatly affect quality of life [64]. Patients with maxillofacial injuries who recounted PTSD symptoms were more likely to also report pre-injury psychological troubles, amplified levels of stress and deprived social support [65].

Furthermore, such patients are also likely to be elder female that experience more injury-related pain [66]. Identification of PTSD signs and symptoms can lead to additional exploration and uncovering of earlier unrecognized psychological symptoms like depression and anxiety disorders [67].

5. Clinical implications of psychological disorders in the injured patient

Injured patients are typically unemployed, socially disadvantaged, mostly males from their mid-twenties to their mid-thirties [48]. They had likely been exposed to prior traumatic events, though they typically did not currently have PTSD from these events at the time of the orofacial injury [48].

With the astronomical rates of unidentified and untreated psychosocial problems in patients suffering from maxillofacial trauma, using the emergency care as a chance to screen for psychosocial troubles will likely increase the discovery of more patients with behavioral disorders that might have precipitated the injury and interfere with a complete recovery. Evidence has shown that psychological assessment of trauma patients followed by referral to mental health services for those identified may result in better aftermath.

Since the acute trauma is frequently the only contact the patients who are healthy young adults have with the hospital, this hospital visit, may offer chances to ascertain psychosocial hitches such as alcohol, drug and substance abuse that may lead to subsequent re-injury and poor treatment outcome. While a substantial subgroup of maxillofacial injuries are associated with alcohol and substance abuse [68], there is potential for integrating brief screening and behavioral interventions into the care of these folks.

Physical scarring and psychological wounds may develop over time, and even become chronic [63]. It is likely that these negative sequelae are going to be even more prevalent in persons who already are experiencing difficulties with substance use, anxiety, depression, hostility, small social networks, limited social support and financial resources, and unmet social service need when they are injured. While surgical treatment may repair the broken bones, many of these patients remain to be at danger for re-injury or deprived psychological outcomes because they may lack the social and personal resources required to make the sustained positive behavior changes. A standard of widespread participation created on the ethics of collective care, wherein medical practitioners from multiple disciplines work together to develop and implement an integrated treatment plan to address the concurrent social and psychologic needs of maxillofacial injury patients is very essential and long overdue [69].

6. Conclusion

Road traffic accident remained the main cause of injury of subject and majorities were males. Most of the patients were young adults. There were significant differences in depression and anxiety level in the maxillofacial injured subjects at baseline

(Time 1), Time 2 (4–8 weeks) and Time 3 (10–12 weeks) with the recording of higher levels of depression and anxiety. Similarly, lower self-esteem was observed subjects at Time 1 (within 1 week), Time 2 (4–8 weeks) and Time 3 (10–12) weeks post injury. The psychological domains of the WHO QoL-Bref was constantly lower than other domains. This shows that maxillofacial injured are psychologically affected apart from the physical injuries they sustained.

7. Recommendations

1. In addition to providing surgical care, the team must be able to address social needs (homelessness, joblessness) and psychological needs (PTSD, depression, anxiety, and substance use).

2. Innovative cost-effective programs which can integrate medical and psychological care are especially necessary in hospitals taking care of trauma patients.

3. Interventions like motivational interviewing which is a brief form of counseling created to assist patients gather personal resources to promote positive behavior change. This can be presented to patients within days of maxillofacial injury and principally important in refining long-term outcomes.

4. Educating surgeons on behavioral issues and offering easily assessable guides for swift screening of psychosocial problems is essential.

5. Developing collaborative bonds with mental health professionals and social health workers are critical first steps regarding incorporating mental health assistances into the full care of maxillofacial injured patients.

6. Studies on psychological aspect of maxillofacial trauma in other continents like Middle East, Asia and African nations should be encouraged for data comparison.

Acknowledgements

My supervisors late professor V.I. Ugboko, Dr. D.I. Ukpong, professor K.C Ndukwe for supervising the project, making several corrections, modifications and suggestions. Many thanks to professor (Mrs) A.O. Fatusi and Dr. S.B. Aregbesola for reading and making corrections. Many thanks also to late professor Olusile and professor F.J. Owotade for their contributions and advice.

Finally, the logistic support provided by the management of Obafemi Awolowo University Teaching Hospitals Complex, Ile-Ife, Nigeria, is gratefully acknowledged.

Conflict of interest

The authors declare no conflict of interest.

Notes

I want to dedicate this work to the following:

To Almighty God, the Beneficent and most Merciful.

To my wife, Engr. (Dr) Mrs. Maryam Niyilola Braimah for her unflinching support and encouragement at all times and my children, Aishah, Aliyah, and Amilah.

And finally to my parents, in-laws, and siblings.

Author details

Ramat Oyebunmi Braimah[1,2*], Dominic Ignatius Ukpong[3] and Kizito Chioma Ndukwe[4]

1 Department of Dental and Maxillofacial Surgery, Usmanu Danfodiyo University Teaching Hospital, Sokoto, Nigeria

2 Department of Oral and Maxillofacial Surgery, Specialty Regional Dental Center, Najran, Kingdom of Saudi Arabia

3 Department of Mental Health, Obafemi Awolowo University/Obafemi Awolowo University Teaching Hospitals Complex, Ile-Ife, Osun State, Nigeria

4 Department of Oral and Maxillofacial Surgery, University of Nigeria, Nsukka, Nigeria

*Address all correspondence to: bunmibraimah@gmail.com

References

[1] Bisson JI, Sheperd JP, Dhutia M. Psychological sequelae of facial trauma. The Journal of Trauma. 1997;**43**:496-500

[2] Levine E, Degutis L, Pruzinsky T, Shin J, Persing JA. Quality of life and facial trauma: Psychological and body image effects. Annals of Plastic Surgery. 2005;**54**:502-510

[3] Cuijpers P, Smit F. Subthreshold depression as a risk factor for major depressive disorder: A review of prospective studies. Acta Psychiatrica Scandinavica. 2004;**109**:325-331

[4] Meningaud JP, Benadiba L, Servant JM, Bertrand JC, Pelicier Y. Depression, anxiety and quality of life: Outcome 9 months after facial cosmetic surgery. Journal of Cranio-Maxillo-Facial Surgery. 2003;**31**:46-50

[5] Bell RB. The role of oral and maxillofacial surgery in the trauma care center. Journal of Oral and Maxillofacial Surgery. 2007;**65**(12):2544-2553

[6] Glynn SM, Asarnow JR, Asarnow R, et al. The development of acute post-traumatic stress disorder after orofacial injury: A prospective study in a large urban hospital. Journal of Oral and Maxillofacial Surgery. 2003;**61**(7):785-792

[7] Bisson JI, Shepherd JP, Joy D, Probert R, Newcombe RG. Early cognitive-behavioural therapy for post-traumatic stress symptoms after physical injury: Randomised controlled trial. The British Journal of Psychiatry. 2004;**184**:63-69

[8] De Sousa A. Psychological issues in oral and maxillofacial reconstructive surgery. The British Journal of Oral & Maxillofacial Surgery. 2008;**46**:661-664

[9] Bhandari M, Jason W, Busse DC, et al. Psychological distress and quality of life after orthopedic trauma: An observational study. Canadian Journal of Surgery. 2008;**51**(1):15-22

[10] Enqvist B, Von konow OL, Bystedt OH. Stress reduction, preoperative hypnosis and perioperative suggestion in maxillofacial surgery: Somatic responses and recovery. Stress Medicine. 1995;**11**:229-233

[11] McGrouther DA. Facial disfigurement. BMJ. 1997;**314**:991-992

[12] Newell R. Psychological difficulties among plastic surgery ex-patients following surgery to the face. British Journal of Plastic Surgery. 2000;**53**:386-392

[13] Le BT, Dierks EJ, Ueeck BA, Homer LD, Potter BF. Maxillofacial injuries associated with domestic violence. Journal of Oral and Maxillofacial Surgery. 2001;**59**:1277-1283

[14] Van Swearingen J. Facial rehabilitation: A neuromuscular reeducation and patient centered approach. Facial Plastic Surgery. 2008;**24**:250-259

[15] Shaikh ZS, Worall SF. Epidemiology of facial trauma in a sample of patients aged 1-18 years. Injury. 2002;**33**:669-671

[16] Thompson A, Kent G. Adjusting to disfigurement: The processes involved in dealing with being visibly different. Clinical Psychology Review. 2001;**21**:663-682

[17] Shepherd JP. Strategies for the study of the long term sequelae of oral and facial injuries. Journal of Oral and Maxillofacial Surgery. 1992;**50**:390-399

[18] Tebble NJ, Thomas DW, Price P. Anxiety and self consciousness in patients with minor facial lacerations. Journal of Advanced Nursing. 2004;**47**:417-426

[19] Sen P, Ross N, Rogers S. Recovering maxillofacial trauma patients: The hidden problem. Journal of Wound Care. 2001;**10**:53-57

[20] Rosenberg M. Society and the Adolescent Self-Image. Princeton, New Jersey: University Press; 1965

[21] Fennell M. Low self-esteem. In: Tarrier N, Wells A, Haddock G, editors. Treating Complex Cases: The Cognitive Behavioural Therapy Approach. London: John Wiley & Sons; 1998

[22] Rahman ZAA, SW Au YL, Ummu AY. The physical and psychological morbidity in maxillofacial trauma patients. Annals of Dentistry University of Malaya. 1999;**6**:8-10

[23] Ukpong DI, Ugboko VI, Ndukwe KC, Gbolahan O. Psychological complications of maxillofacial trauma: A preliminary findings from a Nigerian university teaching hospital. Journal of Oral and Maxillofacial Surgery. 2007;**65**:891-894

[24] Solomon SD, Davidson JRT. Trauma: Prevalence, impairment, service use, and cost. The Journal of Clinical Psychiatry. 1993;**58**(Suppl):5-11

[25] American Psychiatric Association. Diagnostic and Statistical Manual of Mental Disorders: Fourth Edition. Washington DC: American Psychiatric Association; 1994

[26] Yehuda R. Post-traumatic stress disorder. The New England Journal of Medicine. 2002;**346**:108-114

[27] Orr SP, Metzger LJ, Pitman RK. Psychophysiology of post-traumatic stress disorder. The Psychiatric Clinics of North America. 2002;**25**:271-293

[28] Hull AM, Lowe T, Delvin M, et al. Psychological consequences of maxillofacial trauma: A preliminary study. The British Journal of Oral & Maxillofacial Surgery. 2003;**41**:317-322

[29] Bellucci CC, Kapp-Simon KA. Psychological considerations in orthognathic surgery. Clinics in Plastic Surgery. 2007;**34**:11-16

[30] Rumsey N, Harcourt D. Body image and disfigurement: Issues and interventions. Body Image. 2004;**1**:83-97

[31] Haas CF, Champion A, Secor D. Motivational factors for seeking cosmetic surgery: A synthesis of literature. Plastic Surgical Nursing. 2008;**28**:177-182

[32] Kreiger LM, Lee GK. The economics of plastic surgery practices: Trends in income, procedure mix and volume. Plastic and Reconstructive Surgery. 2004;**114**:192-199

[33] Zigmond AS, Snaith RP. The hospital anxiety and depression scale. Acta Psychiatrica Scandinavica. 1983;**67**:361-370

[34] Abiodun OA. A validity study of the hospital anxiety and depression scale in general hospital units and a community sample in Nigeria. The British Journal of Psychiatry. 1994;**165**:669-672

[35] Abiodun OA, Yemisi O. Factors associated with depressive symptoms in Nigerian adolescents. The Journal of Adolescent Health. 2006;**39**:105-110

[36] WHOQOL. The World Health Organization Quality of Life assessment (WHOQOL): Development and general psychometric properties. Social Science and Medicine. 1995;**41**:1403-1409

[37] Olusina AK, Ohaeri JU. Subjective quality of life of recently discharged Nigerian psychiatrist patients. Social Psychiatry and Psychiatric Epidemiology. 2003;**38**:707-714

[38] Brewin CR, Rose S, Andrews B. Brief screening instrument for post-traumatic stress disorder. The British Journal of Psychiatry. 2002;**181**:158-164

[39] Brewin CR. Screening for Post-Traumatic Stress Disorder [Correspondence]. British Journal of Psychiatry. 2002;**181**:535

[40] Lento J, Glynn S, Shetty V, et al. Psychologic functioning and needs of indigent patients with facial injury: A prospective controlled study. Journal of Oral and Maxillofacial Surgery. 2004;**62**:925-932

[41] Fasola AO, Obiechina AE, Arotiba JT. Incidence and pattern of maxillofacial fractures in the elderly. International Journal of Oral and Maxillofacial Surgery. 2003;**32**:206-208

[42] Ugboko VI, Odusanya SA, Fagade OO. Maxillofacial fractures in a semi-urban Nigerian teaching hospital. A review of 442. International Journal of Oral and Maxillofacial Surgery. 1998;**27**:286-289

[43] Oginni FO, Ugboko VI, Ogundipe O, Adegbehingbe BO. Motorcycle related maxillofacial injuries among Nigerian intracity road users. Journal of Oral and Maxillofacial Surgery. 2006;**64**:56-62

[44] Fasola AO, Nyako AE, Obiechina AE, Arotiba JT. Trends in the characteristics of maxillofacial fractures in Nigeria. Journal of Oral and Maxillofacial Surgery. 2003;**61**:1140-1143

[45] Pye G, Waters EA. Effects of seat belt legislation on injuries in road traffic in Nottingham. British Medical Journal. 1984;**288**:756-760

[46] Allen MJ, Barnes MR, Bodiwata GG. The effects of seat belt legislation in injuries sustained by car occupants. Injury. 1985;**16**:471-473

[47] Van Beek GT, Merkx CA. Changes in the pattern of fractures of the maxillofacial skeleton. International Journal of Oral and Maxillofacial Surgery. 1999;**28**:242-248

[48] Glynn S. The psychosocial characteristics and needs of patients presenting with orofacial injury. Oral and Maxillofacial Surgery Clinics of North America. 2010;**22**(2):209-215

[49] Mitchell C. The health impact of intimate partner violence. Journal of the California Dental Association. 2004;**32**:396-398

[50] Ericksson L, Willmar K. Jaw fractures in Malmo 1952-1962 and 1975-1985. Swedish Dental Journal. 1987;**11**:31-36

[51] Oji C. Jaw fractures in Enugu Nigeria, 1985-1995. The British Journal of Oral & Maxillofacial Surgery. 1999;**37**:106-109

[52] McCarthy ML, MacKenzie EJ, Edwin D, LEAP Study Group. Psychological distress associated with severe lower-limb injury. The Journal of Bone and Joint Surgery. American Volume. 2003;**85**:1689-1697

[53] Shepherd JP. Personal violence: The relevance of Symond's model of psychological response and loss theory. British Journal of Social Work. 1990;**1990**(20):309-332

[54] Whetsell LA, Patterson CM, Young DH, Schiller WR. Preinjury psychopathology in trauma patients. The Journal of Trauma. 1989;**29**:1158

[55] Braimah RO, Ukpong DI, Ndukwe KC, Akinyoola AL. Comparative study of anxiety and depression following maxillofacial and orthopedic injuries. Study from a Nigerian university teaching hospital. Clinical and Experimental Dental Research. 2017;**3**:215-219. DOI: 10.1002/cre2.90

[56] Hull AM, Lowe T, Finlay P. The psychological impact of maxillofacial trauma: An overview of reactions to trauma. Oral Surgery, Oral Medicine, Oral Pathology, Oral Radiology, and Endodontics. 2003;**95**:515-520

[57] Park KP, Lim SU, Kim JH, et al. Fracture patterns in the maxillofacial region: A four-year retrospective study. Journal of the Korean Association of Oral and Maxillofacial Surgeons. 2015;**41**(6):306-316

[58] Jackson LA. Physical attractiveness: A sociocultural perspective. In: Cash TF, Pruzinsky T, editors. Body Image: A Handbook of Theory, Research, and Clinical Practice. New York: Guilford Press; 2002. pp. 13-21

[59] Braimah RO, Ukpong DI, Ndukwe KC, Akinyoola AL. Self-esteem following maxillofacial and orthopaedic injuries: Preliminary observations in subSaharan Africans. Oral and Maxillofacial Surgery. 2019;**23**(1):71-76. DOI: 10.1007/s10006-018-0735-5

[60] Mayou R, Bryant B. Outcome in consecutive emergency department attenders following road traffic accidents. The British Journal of Psychiatry. 2001;**179**:528-534

[61] Braimah RO, Ukpong DI, Ndukwe KC, Akinyoola AL. Health-related quality of life in Nigerian patients following maxillofacial and orthopedic injuries: A comparative study. Journal of Orthopaedics, Traumatology and Rehabilitation. 2018;**10**:49-53

[62] Gopalkrishna G, Peek-Asa C, Kraus JF. Epidemiological features of facial injuries among motorcyclists. Annals of Emergency Medicine. 1998;**32**:425-430

[63] Glynn SM, Shetty V, Elliot-Brown K, et al. Chronic post traumatic stress disorder after facial injury: A 1 year prospective cohort study. The Journal of Trauma. 2007;**62**:410-418

[64] Fabio R, Allesandro DA, Guiseppe A, Berrone S. Maxillofacial trauma and psychiatric sequelae: Post traumatic stress disorder. The Journal of Craniofacial Surgery. 2005;**16**:355-360

[65] Herman JL. Complex PTSD: A syndrome in survivors of prolonged and repeated trauma. Journal of Traumatic Stress. 1992;**5**:377-391

[66] Hull AM. Neuroimaging findings in post traumatic stress disorder. The British Journal of Psychiatry. 2002;**181**:102-110

[67] Crowley KE. Aesthetic issues and anxiety management in female oral and maxillofacial surgery patients. Oral and Maxillofacial Surgery Clinics of North America. 2007;**19**:141-152

[68] Murphy DA, Shetty V, Resell J, Zigler C, Yamashita DD. Substance use in vulnerable patients with orofacial injury: Prevalence, correlates, and unmet service needs. The Journal of Trauma. 2009;**66**(2):477-484

[69] Laskin DM. The psychological consequences of maxillofacial injury. Journal of Oral and Maxillofacial Surgery. 1999;**57**(11):1281-1293